D0718618

Diabetes and Cardiovascular Disease

Andrew J Krentz MD, FRCP
Consultant Physician,
Department of Diabetes and Endocrinology,
Southampton University Hospitals, UK

James M Lawrence MBBS, MRCP
Consultant Physician,
Department of Diabetes and Endocrinology,
Salisbury Healthcare NHS Trust, UK

Lucinda KM Summers DPhil, MRCP
Senior Lecturer,
Academic Unit of Molecular Vascular Medicine,
University of Leeds, UK

Ian Walton MBBS, MRCGP
General Practitioner,
Horseley Heath Surgery,
Tipton, West Midlands, UK

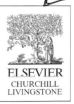

ELSEVIER
CHURCHILL
LIVINGSTONE

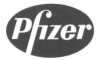

Provided as a Service to Medicine by Pfizer

ISBN 0443 102953
Cataloguing in Publication Data
Catalogue records for this book are available from the US Library of Congress and the British Library.

Note
Knowledge and best practice in this field are constantly changing. As new research and experience broaden our knowledge, changes in practice, treatment and drug therapy may become necessary or appropriate. Readers are advised to check the most current information provided (i) on procedures featured or (ii) by the manufacturer of each product to be administered, to verify the recommended dose or formula, the method and duration of administration, and contraindications. It is the responsibility of the practitioner, relying on their own experience and knowledge of the patient, to make diagnoses, to determine dosages and the best treatment for each individual patient, and to take all appropriate safety precautions. To the fullest extent of the law, neither the Publisher nor the authors assume any liability for any injury and/or damage to persons or property arising out or related to any use of the material contained in this book.

Front cover image of the atherosclerotic plaque reproduced with kind permission of Graham MacGregor, Professor of Cardiovascular Medicine, Blood Pressure Unit, St George's University of London.

Printed in Spain

Acknowledgements

Heidi Harrison, Alison Taylor, Tuan Ho and Rachel Wheeler provided support throughout the preparation of this book. Where not referenced, quotations from authors are reported verbatim from scientific meetings.

AJK was the recipient of a British Heart Foundation International Research Fellowship during part of the writing and editing of this book.

Dedication

To our families.

Contents

Preface

Type 2 diabetes mellitus affects a substantial proportion of the world's population and accounts for >90% of cases of diabetes. As a leading non-communicable disease of modern times diabetes poses a threat to the health of millions of people. The ravages of vascular disease are a key aspect of the public health issues associated with diabetes. Diabetes has an unenviable reputation for causing or exacerbating vasculopathy throughout the circulatory system. So intertwined are type 2 diabetes and cardiovascular disease that it is suggested that they might arise from a shared antecedent: the so-called common soil hypothesis. Obesity and insulin resistance are associated with both diabetes and cardiovascular disease. Moreover, recent clinical trials have shown that some drugs provide protection against cardiovascular events while reducing the risk of developing diabetes.

The aim of this book is to provide an accessible, up-to-date reference for the ever-growing range of health professionals who encounter patients with diabetes. The focus is on primary care, although we discuss aspects of hospital treatment. We have highlighted some areas of controversy, aiming to give a balanced view of current knowledge. From our experience as practising clinicians, we have tried to provide practical guidance about translating a burgeoning evidence base into daily management. Throughout the book, we have endeavoured to give an international perspective. However, it has become impossible to cover the specifics for each country; readers are advised to consult their national guidelines for cardiovascular risk management.

The authors have learned a great deal in the process of writing this book; we hope that readers will find our efforts of some value. In time-honoured fashion, as principal author and editor, I take responsibility for any errors.

Andrew J Krentz
Southampton University Hospitals, UK
Spring 2005

Biographies

Andrew J Krentz MD, FRCP is a consultant physician specializing in diabetes and endocrinology at Southampton University Hospitals, UK. He is honorary senior lecturer at the University of Southampton. Dr Krentz trained in metabolic medicine at the General Hospital, Birmingham, UK and the University of New Mexico, Albuquerque, USA. His clinical and research interests focus on the pathophysiology and management of type 2 diabetes and insulin-resistant states associated with cardiovascular disease. Dr Krentz serves on the editorial boards of several UK and international medical journals. He is an invited member of the European Group for the Study of Insulin Resistance and is a founder member of the International Society of Diabetes and Vascular Disease. In 2004 Dr Krentz was the recipient of a British Heart Foundation International Research Fellowship at the University of California, San Diego, USA. In 2005 Dr Krentz was invited to become a founding member of a new UK group – the Syndrome X Foundation.

James M Lawrence MBBS, MRCP trained at the medical school of St George's Hospital, London, UK, qualifying in 1992. He is currently a consultant physician in diabetes and endocrinology at Salisbury NHS Healthcare Trust, UK, having completed his specialist registrar training in the Wessex region. Dr Lawrence's research interests include diabetes and screening in general practice and lipids and lipoprotein metabolism and macrovascular disease in type 2 diabetes. He has published around 20 original articles, reviews and book chapters on a range of topics including the effects of oral hypoglycaemic agents on lipoprotein subfractions in type 2 diabetes, the effects of high-dose atorvastatin on subfractions, lipids in diabetes, diabetes screening and glitazones and statins.

Lucinda KM Summers DPhil, MRCP trained at King's College, London, UK, qualifying in 1990. She worked in several teaching and district general hospitals in London before accrediting in general medicine, diabetes and endocrinology in 2000. She was a research fellow with the Oxford Lipid Metabolism Group from 1995 to 1998. Since April 2002, Dr Summers has been a senior lecturer in medicine at the University of Leeds, UK, and an honorary consultant specializing in diabetes and general medicine at the General Infirmary, Leeds, UK. She is on the editorial board of the continuing medical education section of *Diabetic Medicine* and has published over 30 original articles, reviews and book chapters on adipose tissue, obesity, insulin resistance and cardiovascular risk. In 2000 she was awarded the Association for the Study of Obesity Young Researcher Award for this work and she continues to have research interests in these areas.

Ian Walton MBBS, MRCGP graduated from the medical school of St Bartholomew's Hospital, London, UK in 1980 and trained as a GP in Staffordshire and New Zealand. He is a GP trainer and teaches medical students. Apart from a sabbatical in Australia, he has worked for 20 years in a group practice in Tipton, one of the most socially deprived boroughs in the UK with some of the highest mortality from coronary heart disease. He is chair of the Tipton Care Organisation, which won an award from Diabetes UK for its Tipton Action for Diabetics (TADpole) project. Dr Walton is coronary heart disease lead for the three Sandwell Primary Care Trusts and a member of the clinical advisory group of the Birmingham and Black Country Cardiac Collaborative. He is also a member of the Birmingham and Coventry Cardiovascular Action Group, which runs educational meetings for primary care professionals and encourages research.

INTRODUCTION

66The diabetes epidemic will continue even if levels of obesity remain constant. Given the increasing prevalence of obesity, it is likely that these figures provide an underestimate of future diabetes prevalence 99
Sarah Wild *et al*, 2001

At the dawn of the 21st century, diabetes presents huge challenges in terms of prevention and management. The vascular complications of diabetes are at the forefront of these concerns.[1] A recent international survey found diabetes to be among the leading modifiable causes of myocardial infarction (MI).[2]

Globally, diabetes mellitus presents enormous and increasingly important public health issues.[3] The prevalence of diabetes for all age groups worldwide was estimated to be 2.8% in 2000 (Figure 1) and 4.4% in 2030. The total number of people with diabetes is projected to rise from 171 million in 2000 to 366 million in 2030. Increasing proportions of deaths from cardiovascular disease (CVD) in less developed countries (Table 1), and increased prevalence and associated consequences of other complications of diabetes are anticipated. Over the past two decades, age-adjusted mortality, especially cardiovascular mortality, has declined in the United States. However, mortality attributable to diabetes has increased sharply, particularly in the last decade. Therefore, patients with diabetes have not experienced the decline in cardiovascular mortality seen in those without diabetes and in the US

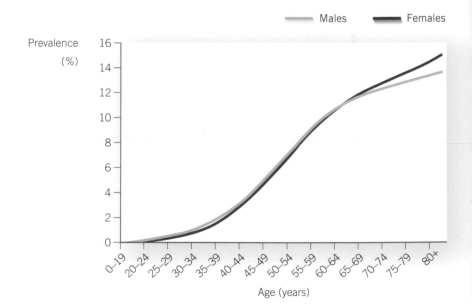

Figure 1. Global diabetes prevalence by age and sex for 2000. Copyright © 2005 American Diabetes Association. From Wild S *et al. Diabetes Care* 2004;27: 1047–1053. Reprinted with permission from *The American Diabetes Association*.

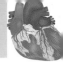

.population at large; this adverse trend is more pronounced for women, in whom mortality rates have been increasing.[4]

The global epidemic of type 2 diabetes, which accounts for around 90% of all cases of diabetes, closely mirrors the explosion in obesity in recent decades (Figures 2 and 3).

	2000		2030	
Ranking	Country	People with diabetes (millions)	Country	People with diabetes (millions)
1	India	31.7	India	79.4
2	China	20.8	China	42.3
3	USA	17.7	USA	30.3
4	Indonesia	8.4	Indonesia	21.3
5	Japan	6.8	Pakistan	13.9
6	Pakistan	5.2	Brazil	11.3
7	Russian Federation	4.6	Bangladesh	11.1
8	Brazil	4.6	Japan	8.9
9	Italy	4.3	Philippines	7.8
10	Bangladesh	3.2	Egypt	6.7

Table 1. List of countries with the highest numbers of estimated cases of diabetes for 2000 and 2030. Copyright © 2005 American Diabetes Association. From Wild S et al. Diabetes Care 2005;27:1047–1053. Reprinted with permission from The American Diabetes Association.

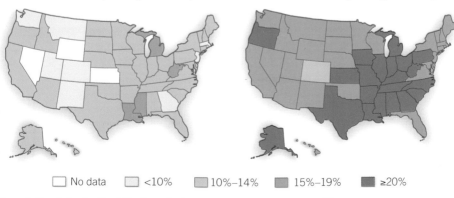

A Prevalence of obesity among US adults, 1991   B Prevalence of obesity among US adults, 2000

☐ No data   ☐ <10%   ☐ 10%–14%   ■ 15%–19%   ■ ≥20%

Figure 2. Trends in obesity, defined as a body mass index ≥30 kg/m², among US adults between 1991 and 2000. Telephone survey of self-reported obesity using random digit dialling. Reproduced from Mokdad AH et al. JAMA 2001;286:1195–1200.

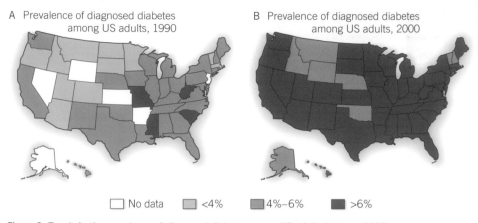

Figure 3. Trends in the prevalence of diagnosed diabetes among US adults between 1990 and 2000. Telephone survey using random digit dialling. Reproduced from Mokdad AH *et al. JAMA* 2001;286:1195–1200.

> *"A pandemic of obesity-related diabetes is in progress"*

Worldwide, obesity is regarded as a major contributor to ill-health.[5] Around 20% of adults in the US, UK and Australia are obese, and this percentage has been steadily increasing. For example, according to data from the Behavioral Risk Factor Surveillance System, 19.8% of the US adult population were obese in 2000.[6] A further 50–60% of US adults are overweight. These figures represent dramatic increases during a single decade (Figure 2).

Obesity is a major modifiable risk factor for diabetes; accordingly, these disorders cluster together (Figure 3). For every kilogram increase in body weight, the risk of diabetes increases by about 5%. Obesity is a leading cause of insulin resistance (see below), which, in turn, may help explain the close associations with diabetes and atherosclerosis. Obesity is regarded as an underlying risk factor for CVD, operating by exacerbating multiple risk factors such as dyslipidaemia, hypertension and inflammation.[7]

> *"Obesity is a major modifiable risk factor for type 2 diabetes and cardiovascular disease"*

In 2000, the prevalence of diagnosed diabetes in the US was 7.3%. According to data from the Third National Health and Nutrition Examination Survey in the US, overweight and obesity are higher in Hispanic men than in non-Hispanic white or black men, and higher in both black and Hispanic women than in non-Hispanic white women. Mexican American boys, together with Mexican American and black girls, have the highest prevalence of overweight, defined as a body

Prevalence (%)*				Table 2. Diabetes trends in the United States from 1995 to 1998 in people older than 18 years.
Ethnic group	**1995**	**1998**	**% Increase**	
White	4.2	4.8	14	
Black	6.5	8.3	28	
Hispanic	4.1	5.1	24	

*Self-reported
Source: http://www.cdc.gov

mass index (BMI) of 25–29 kg/m^2. Between 1995 and 1998, age-adjusted prevalence rates for type 2 diabetes increased strikingly in all ethnic groups in the US (Table 2).[8]

The prevalence of type 2 diabetes has a strong inverse relationship to educational level, but over recent years there have been large increases in the college-educated strata. In 2002, an estimated 6.3% of the US population (around 18 million people) had diabetes with around one-third thought to be undiagnosed.[9]

Total fat consumption has been stable or slightly higher, making up fewer of the total calories consumed overall; carbohydrate intake, as a percentage of total calorie intake, has increased. Of particular concern is the recent emergence of obesity-related type 2 diabetes among adolescents and children; this bodes ill for the long-term prognosis of these individuals who face decades of exposure to major cardiovascular risk factors, often in combination.[10]

In addition to a propensity for microvascular complications – retinopathy, nephropathy and neuropathy – diabetes is associated with an increased risk of atherosclerotic CVD.[1] This is manifested in the:
- Coronary circulation
- Carotid and cerebral arteries
- Peripheral arterial tree.

Moreover, atherosclerosis is responsible for:
- A 30% overall reduction in life expectancy among patients with diabetes
- An annual rate of fatal and non-fatal cardiovascular events among patients with type 2 diabetes of 2–5% in the UK.

DIABETES AND CARDIOVASCULAR DISEASE: AN INTIMATE RELATIONSHIP

Coronary artery disease

Among patients with diabetes, coronary artery disease (CAD) is the leading cause of mortality. Moreover, diabetes is associated with higher mortality rates following MI. The literature suggests increases of up to two-fold compared with non-diabetic patients. The risks of stable angina pectoris and acute coronary syndromes, i.e. sudden death, re-infarction, heart failure and re-stenosis, are appreciably higher in the presence of diabetes.

Population-based studies generally suggest that for patients with type 2 diabetes the relative risk of dying from CAD is increased two- to three-fold in men, and three- to five-fold in women.

66Mortality rates following MI in the patient with diabetes are around twice as high as for people without diabetes 99

Diabetes and cardiovascular disease in women

While the absolute risk of CAD among women with diabetes is similar to that among men, relative risk is higher for women.[11] This eliminates the usual protection enjoyed by females.[12] Adjusting for classic risk factors, i.e. age, hypertension, total cholesterol concentration and smoking, explains much of this effect.[13]

However, the magnitude of risk factor in women with diabetes appears to be more marked than in their male counterparts; the impact of these factors also seems more deleterious. Therefore, post-challenge hyperglycaemia is associated with higher-risk fatal CVD and heart disease in older women.[14] In the Nurses Health Study, a high risk of CVD risk factors was noted before diagnosis of diabetes.[15] The longitudinal Framingham Study in the US demonstrated the higher relative risk of CAD in women with diabetes (Figure 4).[16]

Because CAD is the leading cause of death among women, as it is for men, more research into the impact of cardiovascular risk in women is indicated. Issues such as intrinsic sex-specific differences in pathobiology, late diagnosis of CAD and relative undertreatment of modifiable risk factors, may all be relevant. The associations between polycystic ovary syndrome (PCOS), type 2 diabetes and CVD are discussed later.

The role of hormone replacement therapy (HRT) for post-menopausal women has recently come under intense scrutiny. HRT can improve endothelial function, reduce low-density lipoprotein (LDL) cholesterol concentrations and raise high-density lipoprotein (HDL) cholesterol concentrations.[17] Oestrogen alone has been associated with improvements in surrogate markers for CVD.[17] However, oestrogen can increase C-reactive protein levels (see section on *Cardiovascular risk factors in the patient with diabetes*). Oestrogen-induced inflammation

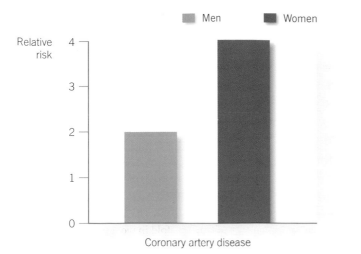

Men Women

Figure 4. Relative risk of coronary artery disease in men and women with diabetes. A relative risk of 1 indicates the relative risk expected in a control group. Adapted from Wilson PWF, Kannel PW. In: Ruderman N *et al.* (eds). *Hyperglycemia, diabetes and vascular disease*. New York: Oxford University Press, 1992; pp. 21–29.

could be a potentially detrimental effect as far as the stability of existing atherosclerotic plaques is concerned.[18]

Two major trials, which used a combination of conjugated equine oestrogen (0.625 mg) and medroxyprogesterone acetate (2.5 mg), did not confirm observational studies suggesting a protective effect. In the Heart and Estrogen/progestin Replacement Study (HERS), there was no overall cardiovascular benefit and a pattern of early increase in risk of coronary events during the first year in women with a history of CAD.[19] The Women's Health Initiative (WHI) was designed to study primary prevention of CVD.[20] Increased risks of stroke and pulmonary emboli were observed. Outcomes between diabetic and non-diabetic women in these trials were similar. Current thinking has moved away from the use of oestrogen–progesterone therapy for prevention of CVD.[21,22]

Among patients of either sex with type 2 diabetes, the risk of death from CAD is further magnified by the presence of microvascular complications, chief among these being diabetic nephropathy (see section on *Cardiovascular risk factors in the patient with diabetes*). The impact of autonomic neuropathy, which is frequently subclinical, has been less well explored but is relevant to aspects of the diagnosis and management of CVD associated with diabetes.

Type 1 diabetes

Type 1 diabetes is characterized by profound insulin deficiency that necessitates insulin replacement therapy. The lifetime risk of CVD in patients with type 1 diabetes is increased. Nephropathy, which develops

13

in around 25–30% of patients with type 1 diabetes, has a particularly close association with atherosclerosis, its presence dramatically increasing the risk of CVD.

"Coronary artery disease is the principal cause of premature mortality in patients with diabetes "

However, clinicians have little information from interventional studies in patients with type 1 diabetes to guide primary preventive therapy. Issues of who to treat with drugs such as statins and angiotensin converting enzyme (ACE) inhibitors, and when to initiate such treatment, need careful assessment of risks and likely benefits. Such considerations are particularly apposite to women with type 1 diabetes in their reproductive years.

Cardiovascular risk factors and diabetes

The importance of diabetes in relation to CAD has become more widely appreciated in recent years. In 2001, the US National Cholesterol Education Panel (NCEP) proposed that diabetes be regarded as a coronary 'risk equivalent'.[23] The impact of diabetes was forcefully demonstrated in a population-based study from Finland. During a seven-year follow-up period, patients with type 2 diabetes who had no overt CAD at entry to the study were found to be at as high a risk of MI and CVD death as people without diabetes who had already sustained an MI (Figure 5).[24] Therefore, many patients with type 2 diabetes may have an absolute risk of MI as high as people without diabetes who have already sustained their first clinical event. Longer follow-up of this cohort has confirmed persistence of the impact of diabetes.

Figure 5. Incidence over a seven-year period of myocardial infarction in people with type 2 diabetes compared with the general population. Note the similarity of risk for non-diabetics with a history of myocardial infarction and people with diabetes with no prior myocardial infarction. Diabetics with a myocardial infarction are at highest risk (CVD = cardiovascular disease; MI = myocardial infarction). Adapted from Haffner SM *et al. N Engl J Med* 1998;339:229–234.

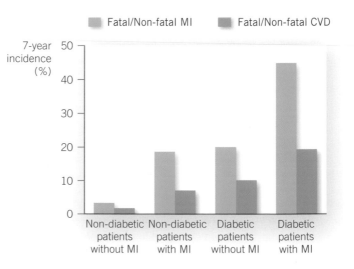

In the general population, the decision to intervene pharmacologically in pursuit of primary prevention has been based on calculating the absolute 10-year risk of cardiovascular events for each individual, 20% being the current threshold. Note that this includes risk of stroke as well as CAD.[25] The current view of the British Hypertension Society (BHS) is that patients with type 2 diabetes aged 50 years or older or whose diabetes has been diagnosed for more than 10 years should be regarded as candidates for measures hitherto reserved for patients with CAD.

Patients with diabetes have been removed from the latest version of the risk prediction charts (www.bhsoc.org). These should not be used for patients with the following conditions that are usually associated with high risk, meriting therapy:

- CAD or other major atherosclerotic disease
- Familial hypercholesterolaemia or other inherited dyslipidaemias
- Chronic renal dysfunction.

In such circumstances, risk is sufficiently high to justify starting drugs to lower blood pressure and LDL-cholesterol levels, where safe and appropriate to do so. No distinction is made between type 1 and type 2 diabetes in the charts; it is suggested that it is reasonable to approach primary prevention in patients older than 40 with type 1 diabetes in an analogous way. Calculating cardiovascular risk in younger patients with type 1 diabetes is problematic.

The high rates of re-infarction (Figures 5 and 6) and generally poor prognosis of patients with diabetes after MI confirmed in recent

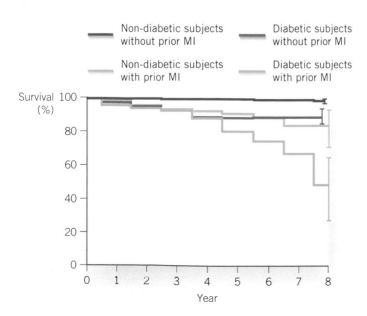

Figure 6. Kaplan–Meier estimates of the probability of death from coronary heart disease in 1059 patients with type 2 diabetes and 1378 non-diabetic patients with and without prior myocardial infarction (MI = myocardial infarction; bars indicate 95% confidence intervals). Reproduced with permission from Haffner S *et al. N Engl J Med* 1998;339:229–234. Copyright © 1998 Massachusetts Medical Society. All rights reserved.

clinical trials[26] support the case for the prevention of coronary artery events. The increased risk of sudden death associated with diabetes strengthens this view. There is still some debate, however.

First, not all studies have confirmed the high risk of MI reported by Haffner *et al*, leading to concerns about unnecessary exposure to drug treatment for some patients. Issues such as selection criteria, i.e. recently diagnosed versus longer duration diabetes, may explain some of the discrepancies between these studies. Second, it has been argued that the results of recent trials of statins in people with type 2 diabetes have not been entirely consistent. Therefore, there is a view that not all patients with type 2 diabetes are at high enough risk of CVD to warrant an indiscriminate approach to statin therapy.[27]

Some populations – for example the Japanese whose background rate of CVD is considerably lower than in the West, and certain groups within Western populations, for example premenopausal women – may have levels of CVD risk that perhaps do not justify statin therapy. For clinicians basing treatment decisions on the risk of the individual patient, the United Kingdom Prospective Diabetes Study (UKPDS) risk engine (www.dtu.ox.ac.uk/riskengine) offers an alternative means to calculate risk for patients with diabetes.[28]

Although aspects of this debate are unresolved, this should not detract from the need to treat aggressively patients who are clearly at high risk of cardiovascular events. Indeed, recent guidelines argue for ever lower LDL-cholesterol targets (see section on *Dyslipidaemia: therapeutic targets*).

Heart failure

Adults with diabetes have a higher risk of heart failure across all age ranges, heart failure being a leading cause of mortality following MI. Factors additional to extensive CAD, for example diabetes-associated cardiomyopathy and autonomic dysfunction, may contribute to this increased risk.[29] The poor prognosis of these patients remains incompletely explained (see section on *Cardiovascular risk factors in the patient with diabetes*).

‟Diabetes confers an increased risk of heart failure ”

Activation of the sympathetic nervous system and the renin–angiotensin system results in deleterious myocardial remodelling. Stimulation of myocardial beta-adrenergic receptors contributes to abnormalities of cellular energy regulation, with a move towards reliance on fatty acids rather than glucose. Heart failure is a risk factor for thromboembolic events, and is often associated with proteinuria and impaired renal function. Insulin resistance is a reported feature of heart failure, even in non-diabetic patients.[30] Moreover, there is evidence that heart failure is associated with an increased risk of developing type 2

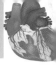

diabetes in the elderly.[31] The clinical implications of insulin resistance in this setting, however, remain unclear.

Cerebrovascular disease

Although less prevalent than CAD, diabetes also confers a higher risk of stroke.[1,32] The incidence of cerebrovascular disease is increased around two- to four-fold in patients with diabetes compared with people without diabetes.

The risk of death from cerebrovascular disease is higher in patients with diabetes, as is the probability of long-term disability. The incidence of transient ischaemic attacks (TIAs) is also increased. Stroke is the second largest cause of death among people with type 2 diabetes.

"The risk of cerebrovascular disease is increased among patients with diabetes"

Peripheral arterial disease

Clinical and subclinical peripheral arterial disease is more common among patients with diabetes.[1] Intermittent claudication is around four times more common in men, and up to six times more common in women with diabetes, compared with age-matched non-diabetic adults. The incidence of distal limb or digital gangrene is greatly increased among patients with diabetes. Arterial disease contributes to the morbidity and mortality associated with diabetic foot disease. In non-diabetic patients the presence of peripheral arterial disease (PAD) denotes a substantially increased risk of cardiovascular events.[33]

"There is a four- to six-fold increase in peripheral vascular disease among patients with diabetes"

CARDIOVASCULAR RISK FACTORS IN THE PATIENT WITH DIABETES

As for the background non-diabetic population, the classic risk factors of hypertension, dyslipidaemia and smoking increase the chances of developing atherosclerosis in patients with diabetes. However, the presence of diabetes powerfully magnifies the impact of these risk factors. Therefore, for any specified level of serum cholesterol, for example, the presence of diabetes confers an additional burden of risk. As risk factors accumulate (see below), the probability of CVD increases steeply (Figure 7).[34,35]

The clinical implication is that thresholds for treating modifiable risk factors, for example hypertension, may need to be lowered for patients with diabetes compared with patients without diabetes. These factors, and others, often cluster together in people more often than would be expected by chance – the collection being known as the "metabolic syndrome" or "syndrome X". The original grouping of risk factors has expanded (Table 3).[36]

The pre-diabetic period, during which risk factors such as hypertension and dyslipidaemia are often present in concert with glucose intolerance and hyperinsulinaemia, has been likened to a "ticking clock" for CVD[37] that starts its countdown years, perhaps decades, before the diagnosis of type 2 diabetes; this may help to explain the high prevalence of atherosclerosis at diagnosis of type 2 diabetes in middle-aged

Figure 7. Panel A. Impact of diabetes on the relationship between serum cholesterol and 10-year mortality from CVD. Panel B. Effects of accumulating risk factors on cardiovascular mortality in diabetic and non-diabetic patients. Adapted from Stamler J et al. *Diabetes Care* 1993;16(2):434–444.

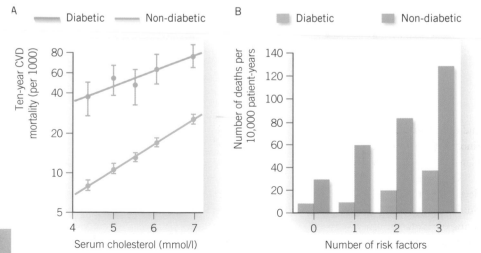

- Glucose intolerance or diabetes*
- Hypertriglyceridaemia*
- Hypertension*
- Impaired insulin-mediated glucose uptake*†
- Decreased HDL cholesterol*
- Small, dense LDL particles; high apolipoprotein B levels
- Abdominal obesity
- Ectopic lipid accumulation in liver and muscle
- Postprandial lipaemia with increased residence time of triglyceride-rich particles
- Hyperuricaemia
- Elevated homocysteine levels
- Elevated serum C-reactive protein levels
- Increased white cell count
- Microalbuminuria (or greater degrees of proteinuria)
- Decreased nitric oxide-dependent vascular endothelial dysfunction
- Increased circulating levels of soluble adhesion molecules

*Original components of Syndrome X as proposed by Reaven
†As measured using the hyperinsulinaemic euglycaemic clamp, a research tool

NB: Not all of these features will be present in every individual with insulin resistance

Table 3. Clinical and biochemical features of the insulin resistance syndrome.

Fibrinogen
Factor VII
Von Willebrand factor
Plasminogen activator inhibitor-1
Tissue plasminogen activator
Factor XIIa

Table 4. Coagulation and fibrinolytic factors linked with cardiovascular disease.

and elderly patients. A pro-thrombotic tendency, allied to impaired fibrinolysis (Table 4), endothelial dysfunction and inflammation, completes the current view of the constellation of adverse vascular threats.

Co-segregation of cardiovascular risk factors may precede the development of type 2 diabetes. A report from the San Antonio Heart Study showed that among people who developed type 2 diabetes, clustering of risk factors for CVD was confined to those with insulin resistance, rather than isolated insulin deficiency (Figure 8).[38]

"The cardiovascular disease risk associated with dyslipidaemia, hypertension or cigarette smoking is amplified by the presence of diabetes"

19

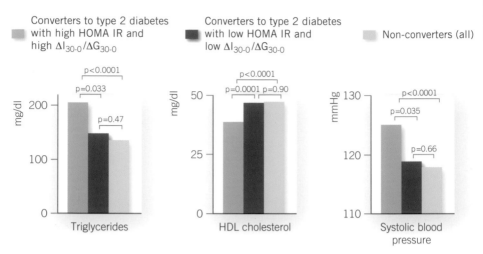

Figure 8. Levels of cardiovascular risk factors by homeostasis model assessment HOMA IR (a surrogate for insulin resistance), a surrogate for insulin secretion ($\Delta I_{30-0}/\Delta G_{30-0}$), and conversion status (to diabetes) (HDL = high-density lipoprotein). Reproduced with permission from Haffner S *et al. Circulation* 2000;101:975–980.

The insulin resistance syndrome

Although diabetes is defined principally by chronic hyperglycaemia, it is complex in its pathophysiology and defects in other aspects of metabolism are usually also present. Citing his own studies and building on contributions from other investigators, Gerald Reaven of Stanford University in the US coined the term syndrome X (also known as the insulin resistance syndrome or Reaven's syndrome) in 1988.[39]

Reaven described the association of insulin resistance, glucose intolerance, dyslipidaemia and hypertension. This clustering is commonly encountered among people with type 2 diabetes. In fact, Reaven inadvertently appropriated the term syndrome X, which was already recognized by cardiologists as so-called microvascular angina in the presence of angiographically normal coronary arteries. Recent studies using intracoronary artery ultrasound suggest that the extent of intramural atheroma may often be underestimated by coronary angiography. Therefore the concept of 'normal' coronary arteries as assessed by contrast angiography is, perhaps, questionable.

While Reaven and others continue to favour the term insulin resistance syndrome, others have opted for the alternatives such as the metabolic syndrome. Notwithstanding semantic considerations, the issue continues to be shrouded in uncertainty and lack of consensus. Major questions surround the concept of the insulin-resistance metabolic syndrome. Is it a syndrome at all? To what extent does a diagnosis of metabolic syndrome improve the prediction of cardiovascular events? Is insulin resistance a fundamental defect? If so, does treatment of insulin resistance *per se* reduce cardiovascular risk?[40]

Risk factor	Defining level	
	Men	**Women**
Waist circumference*	>102 cm (40 inches)	>88 cm (35 inches)
HDL cholesterol	<1.0 mmol/l	<1.3 mmol/l
Fasting triglycerides	≥1.7 mmol/l	≥1.7 mmol/l
Blood pressure	≥130/85 mmHg	≥130/85 mmHg
Fasting venous plasma glucose†	≥6.1 mmol/l	≥6.1 mmol/l

*A measure of central (abdominal) obesity
†A proxy for insulin resistance; this will include patients with type 2 diabetes but will not identify patients with impaired glucose tolerance

Table 5. Diagnosis of the metabolic syndrome according to the National Cholesterol Education Program Adult Treatment Panel III guidelines. The metabolic syndrome is diagnosed in the presence of three or more of these risk factors. Reproduced from Executive Summary of The Third Report of The National Cholesterol Education Program (NCEP) Expert Panel on Detection, Evaluation, and Treatment of High Blood Cholesterol in Adults (Adult Treatment Panel III). *JAMA* 2001;285:2486–2497.

The two leading definitions of the metabolic syndrome have taken somewhat different approaches to diagnosis, perhaps reflecting differences in aims.[41] The World Health Organization (WHO)[42,43] regards insulin resistance as a central component of the syndrome, which predisposes to diabetes and CVD. The NCEP[23] regards the metabolic syndrome as a secondary target for CVD prevention in higher risk patients. The latter definition includes fasting hyperglycaemia as a proxy marker of impaired insulin action (Table 5).

Although both definitions have attracted criticism, they have at least provided a basis for comparing prevalence rates in different populations. However, it is probably fair to say that their impact to date on clinical practice has been limited. Clinicians are faced with a plethora of expert opinions. Alternatives include those of the European Group for the study of Insulin Resistance[44] and the American College of Clinical Endocrinologists.[45]

In addition to some minor differences in thresholds for blood pressure and HDL cholesterol levels, another difference between the WHO and NCEP definitions is the inclusion of microalbuminuria in the former. Although microalbuminuria is a useful marker of increased cardiovascular risk (see the later subsection on *Microalbuminuria*), the nature of its relationship to insulin resistance (Table 3) is less clear.

What is the current prevalence of the metabolic syndrome? A cross-sectional analysis of 8814 men and women aged 20 years or older from the third National Health and Nutrition Examination Survey (1988–1994) revealed prevalence rates ranging from 6.7%, among 20–29 year olds, to 43.5% and 42.0% for those aged 60–69 years and

70 years or older, respectively. The age-adjusted prevalence was 23.7%. Mexican Americans had the highest age-adjusted prevalence of the metabolic syndrome (31.9%).

While the age-adjusted prevalence was similar for men and women, among African Americans, women had about a 57% higher prevalence than men, and among Mexican Americans, women had a 26% higher prevalence than men (Figure 9). Prevalence rates of the metabolic syndrome in European studies have generally been lower (see below).

Studies to date suggest that a diagnosis of the metabolic syndrome confers a two-fold or greater increase in cardiovascular risk. Few studies have examined the impact of the metabolic syndrome on mortality. Using a modification of the WHO criteria, a study of non-diabetic middle-aged European patients found that the metabolic syndrome was associated with an increased risk of all-cause and cardiovascular mortality over a median follow-up period of around nine years.[46] The age-standardized prevalence of the metabolic syndrome was slightly higher in men (15.7%) than in women (14.2%). The overall hazard ratios for all-cause and cardiovascular mortality in patients with the metabolic syndrome, compared with those without it, were 1.44 and 2.26 in men and 1.38 and 2.78 in women after adjustment for age, blood cholesterol levels and smoking.

The cut-offs for waist circumference in the NCEP definition have generated debate. For susceptible individuals or groups, notably South and East Asians, lesser accumulations of abdominal fat can precipitate

Figure 9. Age-adjusted prevalence of the metabolic syndrome among 8814 US adults aged 20 years or older, by sex, race or ethnicity. Reproduced from Ford E *et al. JAMA* 2002;287:356–359.

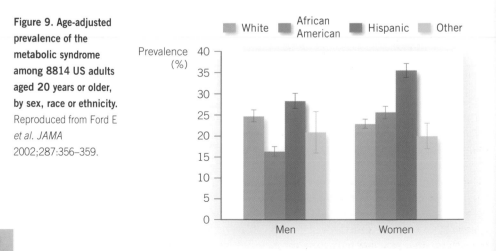

or aggravate metabolic cardiovascular risk factors; this is not reflected in the diagnostic criteria. Even with the generous waist circumference – a marker for central obesity – allowed by the NCEP criteria, the metabolic syndrome is highly prevalent in the US, with nearly 50 million being affected.[47] In an appraisal of waist circumference used as a proxy marker of abdominal obesity, Reaven has pointed out the many protocols that have been applied in various studies. The strong correlation between waist circumference and BMI leads Reaven to suggest using BMI in clinical practice.

For patients with diabetes, the presence of the metabolic syndrome appears to be an important determinant of cardiovascular risk. In a recent study, if diabetes was present in the absence of the metabolic syndrome defined using NCEP criteria, the prevalence of CAD was not increased.[48] The highest risk was seen in those with diabetes and the metabolic syndrome (Figure 10). This study may have underestimated the risks associated with the metabolic syndrome through the phenomenon of 'survivor effect'.

"The thresholds defining the clinical implications of generalized and central obesity are lower in some ethnic groups"

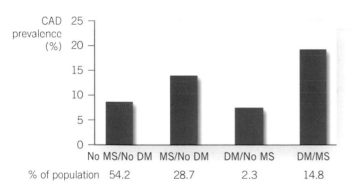

Figure 10. Age-adjusted prevalence of coronary artery disease in the US population older than 50 years categorized by the presence of metabolic syndrome and diabetes. Combinations of metabolic syndrome (MS) and diabetes mellitus (DM) status are shown. Copyright © 2003 American Diabetes Association. From *Diabetes* 2003;52:1210–1214. Reprinted with permission from *The American Diabetes Association*.

	No MS/No DM	MS/No DM	DM/No MS	DM/MS
% of population	54.2	28.7	2.3	14.8

CAD prevalence (%) axis: 0, 5, 10, 15, 20, 25

What is the role of insulin resistance?

Insulin resistance is considered to be present when the actions of insulin elicit a quantitatively subnormal biological response.[49] Insulin binds with high affinity to specific transmembrane receptors. This initiates a complex cascade of intracellular events that culminate in acute metabolic and longer-term mitogenic effects. Most often, insulin resistance has been regarded as an impaired ability of insulin to stimulate the uptake and disposal of glucose in target tissues. However, this approach, which in any case can be performed only in a clinical research environment, may not necessarily reflect the actions of insulin

"Insulin resistance is a plague of the 21st century"
Gerald Reaven, 2004

23

"There is no method for measuring insulin resistance in routine clinical practice"

on other aspects of metabolism, such as on lipoproteins or the regulation of autonomic, vascular and platelet function.

There is a wide range of insulin sensitivity even among otherwise healthy people with normal glucose tolerance. Insulin resistance is common in people with:

- Obesity
- Type 2 diabetes
- Impaired glucose tolerance.

Around 30% of unselected, apparently healthy populations have insulin resistance comparable with that encountered in patients with type 2 diabetes.

Whole body insulin sensitivity is determined by genetic and environmental factors, including abdominal obesity, skeletal muscle mass and physical activity levels. Whether visceral fat accumulation is a primary driver of insulin resistance remains uncertain, although theoretical considerations of increased rates of lipolysis and other metabolic defects make for an attractive hypothesis. It should, however, be emphasized that insulin resistance does not cause obesity.

Recent studies have drawn attention to the role of so-called ectopic fat deposition in liver and muscle in relation to whole body insulin resistance.[50] Non-alcoholic fatty liver disease (NAFLD) is a potentially serious long-term feature of insulin resistance, which presents primarily to hepatologists. Chronic steatohepatitis, in which fat deposition in the liver is complicated by inflammation and fibrosis, occurs in a subgroup of patients with NAFLD.[51]

The maintenance of normal glucose metabolism relies on the following events occurring in a closely regulated manner:

- Insulin secretion – stimulated primarily by hyperglycaemia
- Suppression of gluconeogenesis, mainly hepatic, by hyperglycaemia and hyperinsulinaemia
- Glucose uptake by peripheral tissues – mainly skeletal muscle – stimulated by hyperglycaemia and hyperinsulinaemia
- Glucose uptake by splanchnic tissues – mainly liver – stimulated by hyperglycaemia.

"Around 30% of apparently healthy people have appreciable degrees of insulin resistance"

The effect of insulin on hepatic gluconeogenesis and on muscle glucose uptake is much greater than the mass action effect of hyperglycaemia. The relevance of insulin resistance to the development of specific cardiovascular risk factors is considered in more detail in other chapters. Impaired insulin action is a feature of many apparently diverse disorders (Table 6); cause and effect relationships are often unclear.

There is currently no way of readily measuring insulin action in clinical practice. Therefore, the presence of insulin resistance is imperfectly inferred from the presence of other clinical or biochemical features.

Table 6. Disorders found in association with insulin resistance.

Lifestyle factors (NB: may be influenced by genetic or intrauterine factors)*
• Obesity, especially abdominal or upper body • Type 2 diabetes and states of glucose intolerance • Physical inactivity
Medical emergencies (increased concentrations of counter-regulatory hormones and cytokines)*
• Acute myocardial infarction • Severe sepsis • Trauma • Diabetic ketoacidosis
Endocrinopathies
• Thyrotoxicosis* • Polycystic ovary syndrome† • Acromegaly‡ • Cushing's syndrome‡ • Phaeochromocytoma‡ • Insulinoma§ • Glucagonoma§
Major organ failure†
• Congestive cardiac failure • Hepatic cirrhosis • Chronic renal failure
Inherited‡ or §
• Myotonic dystrophy • Prader-Willi syndrome • Alstrom's syndrome • Laurence-Moon-Biedl syndrome • Friedreich's ataxia • Syndromes of extreme insulin resistance
Drug therapy*
• Corticosteroids – dose-dependent effects • Beta-blockers, particularly non-selective drugs • Thiazide, thiazide-like and loop diuretics, at high doses • Protease inhibitors
Miscellaneous
• Cystic fibrosis† • Klinefelter's syndrome‡ • Turner's syndrome‡
*Common; †relatively common; ‡uncommon; §rare

"Insulin resistance is associated with obesity, in particular, with increased visceral or upper body fat deposition"

Patients with obesity, the dermatological marker acanthosis nigricans (a hyperpigmented lesion often seen in the axillae or the nape of the neck) or PCOS, together with most patients with type 2 diabetes, are assumed to be insulin resistant.[49] Note, however, that a small proportion of obese people maintain near-normal insulin sensitivity. Measuring fasting plasma insulin concentrations on an individual basis is of limited use, because of lack of standardization between laboratories and absence of accurate reference ranges.

Polycystic ovary syndrome

PCOS usually presents with symptoms of hyperandrogenism, i.e. hirsutism, acne or androgenic alopecia in the second and third decades of life. The syndrome is common – some 5–10% of women of reproductive age are thought to be affected in the US – but the absence of a universally agreed definition is an obstacle to prevalence studies. Oligomenorrhoea is a prominent feature but is not invariable. A history of previous weight gain is common. More than 50% of affected women are obese, abdominal adiposity being the rule even in overweight women. However, there is considerable variability. Somewhat paradoxically, the presence of polycystic ovaries on ultrasound imaging is not a prerequisite for the diagnosis of PCOS.

"Some 5–10% of women of reproductive age are thought to have PCOS in the US"

Most affected women have features of the insulin resistance syndrome, including dyslipidaemia and non-traditional risk markers such as elevated levels of inflammatory markers;[52,53] hyperinsulinaemia is the rule, the impairment of insulin action being in excess of that expected for the degree of adiposity. Women with oligomenorrhoea tend to have the most severe defects in insulin action. Affected women are at increased risk of developing type 2 diabetes, now regarded as a CAD risk equivalent (see above). Expert groups such as the American Association of Clinical Endocrinologists suggest that women with PCOS be screened for diabetes from the age of 30 years, and modifiable cardiovascular risk factors be identified and treated (www.aace.com/clin/guidelines). In fact, there is little firm epidemiological evidence of an excess of CVD events in women with PCOS.

Management is directed towards the primary symptoms, but includes attention to cardiovascular risk factors. Weight reduction is best achieved through diet and exercise where possible. Loss of excess adiposity reduces circulating insulin levels reflecting improved whole body insulin sensitivity. Levels of ovarian androgen decline. Ovulation rates tend to improve although antioestrogen therapy with clomifene citrate may be needed.

Adjunctive drug therapy for hyperandrogenism includes the biguanide metformin (see section on *Prevention and treatment: current and emerging strategies*) and, experimentally, thiazolidinediones (see section on *Prevention and treatment: current and emerging strategies*). These drugs have insulin-sensitizing properties that are exploited in the treatment of type 2 diabetes; however, neither class is licensed for use in PCOS in the absence of diabetes. A recent review concluded that metformin is an effective treatment for anovulation in PCOS.[54] There is some evidence of benefit of metformin on aspects of the metabolic syndrome. However, no data are available regarding the safety of metformin in long-term use in younger women, and only limited data exist concerning its safety in early pregnancy.

Syndromes of extreme insulin resistance

Very rarely, insulin resistance is associated with pseudo-acromegaly in the presence of normal growth hormone and insulin-like growth factor-1 (IGF-1) concentrations. Uncommon congenital or acquired forms of lipodystrophy are also associated with insulin resistance and diabetes (Table 7). These examples of extreme degrees of insulin resistance, which are unlikely to be encountered outside specialist centres, can be difficult to treat; massive doses of insulin may be needed.[55]

Insulin receptor mutations

- Leprechaunism – severe growth retardation is a major feature; usually fatal in infancy
- Rabson-Mendenhall syndrome – rare; may survive into second or third decade of life
- Type A insulin resistance – often not obese. Appears to overlap with polycystic ovary syndrome; marked hyperandrogenism is characteristic in females. Other insulin-resistant patients with obesity, hyperandrogenism, insulin resistance and acanthosis nigricans (HAIR-AN syndrome) may not have mutations in the insulin receptor

Post-binding defects in insulin action, i.e. intracellular signalling defects

- Congenital generalized lipodystrophy (Berardinelli-Seip syndrome)
- Partial lipodystrophy (due to mutation in gene coding for lamin A/C)
- Acquired lipodystrophy (secondary to some anti-retroviral therapies)
- Type C insulin resistance

Insulin receptor antibodies

- Type B insulin resistance

Table 7. Syndromes of extreme insulin resistance. All these syndromes are uncommon or rare. Compensatory hyperinsulinaemia may be sufficient to overcome the defect and glucose tolerance, therefore, may be relatively normal. Overall, morbidity and mortality tend to be high.

Recombinant IGF-1 and leptin, a peptide produced by adipocytes, have been used with some success in a few patients with lipoatrophy.[56]

An interesting feature of some of the lipodystrophy syndromes is the development of cirrhosis. This possibly represents the end-stage of chronic steatohepatitis (see above). Another adipocytokine, adiponectin, has attracted interest as a possible link between obesity, insulin resistance and CVD (Figure 11). Not only does adiponectin, which has similarities to collagen, improve insulin action, it reduces inflammation within the vasculature. Chronic inflammation is thought to be an important component of atherosclerosis, which is reflected in increases in C-reactive protein levels as measured using high-sensitivity assays (see above). In contrast to leptin, circulating levels of adiponectin are low in people with insulin resistance, but can be increased by the insulin-sensitizing thiazolidinedione class of drugs (see section on *Prevention and treatment: current and emerging strategies*).[57]

Recent interest has focused on a more common form of lipodystrophy encountered in patients receiving protease inhibitors for acquired

Figure 11. Actions of adiponectin in skeletal muscle. Adiponectin increases activity of the insulin receptor. It also increases free (non-esterified) fatty acid (FFA) oxidation with reduced intramyocellular triglyceride (TG) accumulation in the liver. The decreased free fatty acid influx and increased oxidation contribute to reduced hepatic glucose output and very-low-density lipoprotein triglyceride synthesis in vascular endothelium. Adiponectin decreases monocyte adhesion to endothelium, suppresses macrophage to foam cell transformation, and inhibits vascular smooth muscle cell proliferation and migration. Copyright © 2003 American Diabetes Association. From *Diabetes Care* 2003;26:2442–2450. Reprinted with permission from *The American Diabetes Association*.

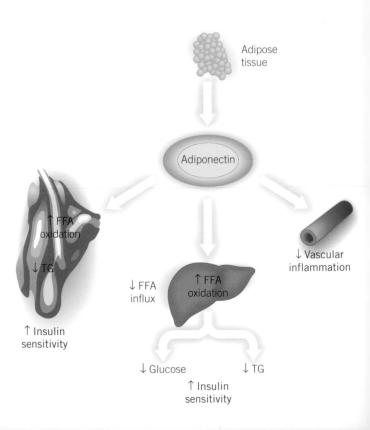

immune deficiency syndrome (AIDS). Associated metabolic abnormalities include dyslipidaemia, insulin resistance and glucose intolerance; an increased incidence of cardiovascular events has been reported.[58]

Limited data in monogenic forms of extreme insulin resistance provide support for an increased frequency of cardiovascular events.[59] Of much more relevance from a public health perspective, certain populations appear to be intrinsically more susceptible to insulin resistance, albeit to a lesser degree than is typical of the rare insulin resistance syndromes. These populations include:

- North American Indians, for example the Pima Indians of Arizona
- Pacific Islanders, for example the Nauruans
- Australian Aborigines
- South Asians.

The prevalence of diabetes is highest among some of these populations, the Pima Indians having the highest risk. The molecular basis for the differences between populations is largely unexplained. In 1962, Neel proposed the 'thrifty genotype' hypothesis.[60] In prehistory, when food supplies were precarious, it was argued, genes conferring metabolic efficiency were selected and these became highly prevalent in many populations. Later, when people could control their food supply, the same genes became detrimental because of their propensity for causing insulin resistance and type 2 diabetes.

It is not certain whether type 2 diabetes is the product of environmental interactions with relatively few potent genes, or with larger numbers of less powerful gene products. Not surprisingly, unravelling the genetics of type 2 diabetes has proved a challenge. The Barker–Hales 'thrifty phenotype' hypothesis proposes that suboptimal intrauterine nutrition may predispose to insulin resistance, diabetes and CVD in adulthood.[61] The risks are highest with excessive weight gain.

Certain stages of life are associated with relative insulin insensitivity which, in the absence of diabetes, usually remains subclinical:

- During puberty, secondary to secretion of hormones that antagonize the metabolic actions of insulin
- During the second and third trimester of pregnancy. Progesterone, cortisol, prolactin, human placental lactogen and oestrogen have been shown in animal models to influence insulin secretion and/or tissue sensitivity to insulin.

The effect of age on insulin sensitivity has been disputed. Some studies suggest insulin resistance increases with age. There is a tendency towards lower activity levels and loss of lean tissue (sarcopenia) with advancing years. The postmenopausal state is associated with adverse changes in body composition and insulin sensitivity.

> *Certain physiological states are associated with transient insulin resistance*

As long as the insulin-producing β-cells of the pancreatic islets are not unduly compromised, insulin resistance is usually accompanied by compensatory hyperinsulinaemia that maintains normal glucose tolerance. There has been a long-running debate as to whether, under these circumstances, hyperinsulinaemia has direct adverse effects on atherogenesis.[62] Epidemiological studies have produced conflicting results, partly reflecting methodological issues. A meta-analysis concluded that hyperinsulinaemia *per se* was a relatively weak predictor of CVD.[63] Similar results were found in a more recent meta-analysis of data from these investigators. This showed that hyperinsulinaemia, defined by the highest quartile cut-off for fasting insulin, was significantly associated with cardiovascular mortality in both men and women independently of other risk factors. Associations between high two-hour postchallenge insulin and cardiovascular mortality were weaker.[64]

In fact, recent clinical trials have shown improved measures of vascular function in patients with type 2 diabetes treated with exogenous insulin.[65] On balance, we take the view that timely insulin treatment has cardiovascular benefits that outweigh disadvantages such as weight gain.[66] Taken together with the metabolic benefits of insulin, we suggest that this evidence should take precedence over the aforementioned theoretical concerns. In this regard, it is important to understand that in the presence of insulin resistance, hyperinsulinaemia may nonetheless be accompanied by a relative deficiency of insulin action within target cells.

This brings us to another aspect of the debate: whether a dichotomy can exist between the impaired effects of insulin on glucose metabolism and production of endothelial nitric oxide, and the deleterious mitogenic and pro-atherogenic pathways that may be stimulated by the presence of high insulin levels (Figure 12). Whether the results of in vitro studies that support this contention are relevant to the situation in vivo is uncertain.

Endothelial dysfunction is regarded as an important early precursor of atherosclerosis in non-diabetic and diabetic patients.[67] Classic and non-traditional risk factors are associated with endothelial dysfunction leading to impairment of nitric oxide release, increased oxidative stress, and loss of protection against atherosclerosis (Figure 13).

Insulin resistance in patients with type 1 diabetes is generally held to be reversible with adequate insulin replacement therapy. Excess adiposity or other acquired causes of insulin resistance, for example

"The role of insulin in the development and progression of cardiovascular disease is controversial"

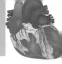

high-dose corticosteroid therapy for related autoimmune disease, may necessitate higher doses of insulin, as may puberty and pregnancy (see above). The development of diabetic nephropathy or heart failure may be associated with exacerbation of insulin resistance.

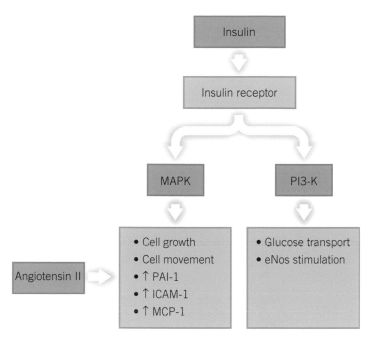

Figure 12. Metabolic and mitogenic pathways of insulin action. Impaired insulin action in the PI3-kinase pathway leads to compensatory hyperinsulinaemia; if the resulting high insulin levels activate the MAP-kinase pathway, this might stimulate mitogenesis in vascular smooth muscle and adhesion of monocytes. Other deleterious factors such as angiotensin II might aggravate the process (eNos = endothelial nitric oxide synthase; ICAM-1 = intracellular adhesion molecule-1; MAPK = mitogen activated protein kinase; MCP-1 = monocyte chemoattractant protein-1; PAI-1 = plasminogen activator inhibitor-1; PI3-K = phosphatidylinositol 3-kinase). Reprinted from Hsueh WA, Quinones MJ. *Am J Cardiol* 2003;92(4A):10J–17J with permission from Excerpta Medica, Inc.

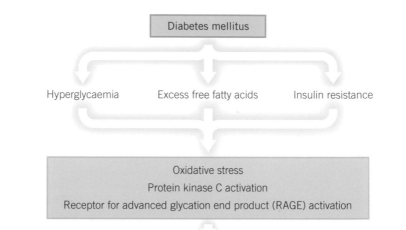

Diabetes mellitus

Hyperglycaemia   Excess free fatty acids   Insulin resistance

Oxidative stress
Protein kinase C activation
Receptor for advanced glycation end product (RAGE) activation

Endothelium

↓ Nitric oxide	↓ Nitric oxide	↓ Nitric oxide
↑ Endothelin-1	↑ Activation of NF-κB	↑ Tissue factor
↑ Angiotensin II	↑ Angiotensin II	↑ Plasminogen activator inhibitor-1
	↑ Activation of activator protein-1	↓ Prostacyclin

Vasoconstriction

- Hypertension
- Vascular smooth muscle cell growth

Inflammation

- Release of chemokines
- Release of cytokines
- Expression of cellular adhesion molecules

Thrombosis

- Hypercoagulation
- Platelet activation
- Decreased fibrinolysis

Atherogenesis

Figure 13. In diabetes, hyperglycaemia, excess non-esterified (free fatty acids) and insulin resistance impair endothelial function, augment vasoconstriction, increase inflammation and promote thrombosis. Decreasing nitric oxide and increasing endothelin-1 and angiotensin II concentrations increase vascular tone and vascular smooth muscle cell growth and migration. Activation of the transcription factors nuclear factor B (NF-κB) and activator protein-1 induces inflammatory gene expression, with liberation of leukocyte-attracting chemokines, increased production of inflammatory cytokines, and augmented expression of cellular adhesion molecules. Increased production of tissue factor and plasminogen activator inhibitor-1 creates a prothrombotic milieu, while decreased endothelium-derived nitric oxide and prostacyclin favours platelet activation. Reproduced with permission from *JAMA* 2002;287:2570–81. Copyright © 2002, *American Medical Association*. All rights reserved.

Hyperglycaemia

Hyperglycaemia is the biochemical hallmark of diabetes. However, the links between hyperglycaemia and excess CVD remain incompletely delineated. Chronic elevations of blood glucose reflect insulin deficiency or, as in the case of most patients with type 2 diabetes, a combination of relative insulin deficiency and impaired insulin action (Figure 14).[68] Both defects are logical targets for therapeutic intervention.

Increases in fasting plasma glucose concentration are closely related to increases in basal hepatic glucose production. Hepatic glucose production in the postabsorptive period (when all of the last meal has been absorbed from the intestinal tract, typically during the fasting period overnight) is within the normal range in people with impaired glucose tolerance because hyperinsulinaemia overcomes hepatic insulin resistance. Fasting hyperglycaemia develops when hepatic glucose production is not adequately suppressed, although absolute rates of glucose production by the liver need not necessarily be elevated. Impaired suppression of hepatic glucose production also makes an important contribution to postprandial hyperglycaemia.[69] Accelerated rates of lipolysis, resulting from insulin resistance in adipocytes, may cause secondary metabolic defects in skeletal muscle and liver. Chronic elevations of glucose and fatty acids can impair islet β-cell function; these toxic effects are known as glucotoxicity and lipotoxicity, respectively.

66The epidemiological evidence linking diabetes with cardiovascular morbidity and mortality is such that no example in the medical literature – other perhaps than smoking and lung cancer – is so strong 99
Ele Ferrannini, 2004

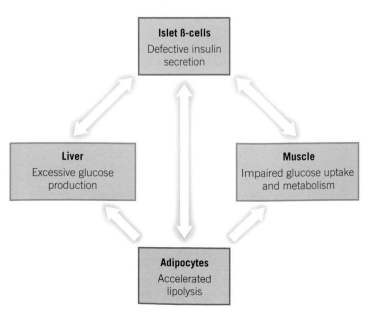

Figure 14. The main tissues involved in regulation of glucose metabolism. Complex defects in multiple cellular biochemical pathways conspire to produce the type 2 diabetes phenotype. The arrows indicate the major interactions between tissues. The primacy of the defects, i.e. impaired insulin action versus defective insulin secretion has not been determined. The relative importance of these defects may differ between people and change with time and treatment.

"Insulin resistance is a prominent metabolic defect in type 2 diabetes"

In most people with type 2 diabetes, muscle glucose disposal in response to insulin infusion is decreased by up to 50%, as determined by clinical investigators using the glucose clamp technique (see section on *Diabetes and cardiovascular disease: an intimate relationship*). Having said this, there is perhaps more heterogeneity between people in terms of insulin resistance than is often assumed. In people without diabetes, about two-thirds of the glucose taken up by muscle is converted to glycogen and stored for future use. The remaining third undergoes oxidation to produce immediate energy sources, such as adenosine triphosphate. Both processes are impaired in type 2 diabetes.

The relative contributions of genetic inheritance, fetal programming and acquired muscle insulin resistance, for example to excess availability of fatty acids (which compete with glucose for uptake and metabolism) or to intramyocellular lipid deposition, are uncertain. In skeletal muscle, insulin resistance is associated with defects at multiple postreceptor sites. Insulin binds to a receptor, consisting of two α- and two β-subunits, at the cell membrane (Figure 12). The number of receptors and their binding affinity are normal or slightly diminished in patients with impaired glucose tolerance or type 2 diabetes. Insulin binds to the α-subunits and transmits its signal to the β-subunits, resulting in phosphorylation of specific tyrosine residues. This activates a cascade of phosphorylation–dephosphorylation reactions that enable glucose to be transported into the cell.

In muscle, the facilitative glucose transporter GLUT-4 is found in vesicles within the cytoplasm. GLUT-4 is one of a family of glucose transporters, not all of which are regulated by insulin. These vesicles are translocated to the cell surface and inserted into the membrane in response to insulin.[70] Once GLUT-4 is activated by insertion into the membrane, glucose is transported into the cell and phosphorylated by hexokinase II to form glucose-6-phosphate (Figure 15).[70] In turn, glucose-6-phosphate is either oxidized or converted to glycogen. With the exception of rare cases of extreme insulin resistance (see section on *Syndromes of extreme insulin resistance*), determining which of these defects are primarily responsible for common forms of insulin resistance has proved difficult. Rapid changes in GLUT-4 expression occur in response to exercise.

Mechanisms of vascular damage

Several potential pathogenic mechanisms suggest a causal relationship between hyperglycaemia and vascular disease. Hyperglycaemia leads to:
- Accelerated formation of advanced glycation end products (AGE)
- Formation by AGE of irreversible abnormal deposits in the subintimal layers of blood vessels

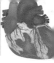

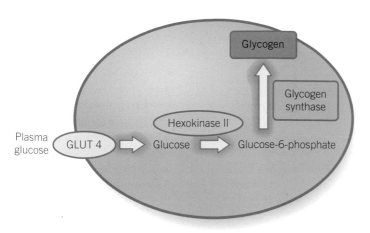

Figure 15. Potential rate-controlling steps responsible for reduced insulin-stimulated muscle glycogen synthesis in patients with type 2 diabetes mellitus. Modified from *J Clin Invest* 2000;106(2):171–176.

- Interference by these deposits with cellular interactions and generation of toxic reactive oxygen species
- Modification of LDL particles through glycation, rendering them more susceptible to oxidation
- Thickening and leakage of the vasculature due to cross-linking of vascular proteins by AGE
- Activation of protein kinase-C leading to increased vascular permeability
- Activation of the polyol pathway with secondary cellular osmotic and ionic changes.

The receptor for AGE is expressed by vascular endothelial and smooth muscle cells, macrophages, monocytes, cardiac myocytes, and neuronal and mesangial cells, and mediates some of these effects. Receptor expression is upregulated in arterial atherosclerotic tissue from people with diabetes. The glycation product receptor interaction in the endothelium leads to upregulation of:

- Plasminogen activator inhibitor-1
- Tissue factor
- Vascular cell adhesion molecule-1 (VCAM-1).

VCAM-1 is expressed on the endothelium in atherosclerotic plaques and causes increased monocyte adhesion. Chemotaxis at sites of AGE accumulation recruits monocytes expressing receptors, where they infiltrate subendothelial layers of the vessels to form foam cells. Other ligands for these receptors include a member of the S100 protein family. Other members of this family are found in atherosclerotic plaques and exert chemoattractant effects on mononuclear phagocytes.

Ligand–receptor interaction induces expression on endothelial cells, mononuclear phagocytes and lymphocytes of:

- Tumour necrosis factor-α (TNF-α)
- VCAM-1
- Interleukin-1.

All these factors are involved in formation of atheromatous plaques. Several polymorphisms in the AGE receptor gene have been identified. The Gly82Ser polymorphism results in inflammation. These changes could potentially lead to the development of vascular disease. It has been suggested that exogenous glycation products derived from fatty foodstuffs may contribute to vascular damage. Renal failure reduces excretion of AGE.[71]

Diagnosis of diabetes and glucose intolerance

Diabetes is readily diagnosed in people with typical osmotic symptoms or specific microvascular complications. In these circumstances, a single venous plasma glucose measurement is usually sufficient. However, the situation is often more complicated because many people with chronic glucose intolerance or type 2 diabetes are asymptomatic. When patients present with a coronary event after many years of unrecognized hyperglycaemia, they may already have significant vascular damage by the time they are diagnosed with diabetes (see section on *Diabetes and cardiovascular disease: an intimate relationship*). Clinicians should therefore retain a high index of suspicion in patients with:

- Obesity, especially abdominal or upper body adiposity
- A personal history of glucose intolerance or diabetes, e.g. gestational diabetes
- A first-degree family history of diabetes.

Treatment with diabetogenic drugs, the presence of atherosclerotic disease or other components of the metabolic syndrome (see section on *Diabetes and cardiovascular disease: an intimate relationship*) should also prompt testing for diabetes. The importance of ethnicity has already been discussed.

"The American Diabetes Association diagnostic criteria for diabetes are based predominantly on fasting blood glucose concentrations"

The American Diabetes Association (ADA)[72] defines diabetes as a fasting plasma glucose concentration ≥ 7.0 mmol/l. Unlike the WHO, the ADA does not generally recommend using a glucose tolerance test (Table 8).[43] Although the fasting plasma glucose has the advantage of being practical, it is less sensitive for detecting diabetes and, by definition, cannot diagnose impaired glucose tolerance (IGT).

Impaired glucose tolerance is associated with an increased risk of CVD. Some studies have shown that people with IGT are more insulin resistant than those with isolated fasting hyperglycaemia.[73] This may be relevant to the association between post-challenge

Category	Criteria
Type 2 diabetes	**With symptoms of diabetes** Random venous plasma glucose ≥11.1 mmol/l OR Fasting plasma glucose ≥7.0 mmol/l **Without symptoms of diabetes** Two plasma glucose results in the diabetic range on different days OR 2-hour plasma glucose concentration ≥11.1 mmol/l 2 hours after 75 g oral glucose tolerance test
Impaired glucose tolerance	Fasting plasma glucose <7.0 mmol/l and ≥7.8 mmol/l but <11.1 mmol/l 2 hours after 75 g oral glucose tolerance test
Impaired fasting glucose	Fasting plasma glucose ≥5.6 mmol/l but <7.0 mmol/l Oral glucose tolerance test recommended to confirm diagnosis (2-hour value)

Table 8. Diagnostic criteria for type 2 diabetes, impaired glucose tolerance and impaired fasting glucose. Data taken from American Diabetes Association, 2004. Diagnosis and classification of diabetes mellitus. *Diabetes Care* 2004;27(Suppl):S5–S10.

hyperglycaemia and cardiovascular mortality (see below). The rate of progression from impaired glucose tolerance to type 2 diabetes is around 5–10% per year, depending on factors such as age and ethnicity.

Diabetes and cardiovascular risk

Epidemiological studies suggest there is a linear association between mean glycated haemoglobin concentration and CVD in patients with type 2 diabetes. For example, in a prospective population-based study of elderly patients in Finland, the 10-year risk of cardiovascular mortality was linearly associated with the tertile of glycaemia at baseline; this association was independent of antidiabetic therapy, i.e. diet, oral antidiabetic drugs or insulin.[74] In another Finnish study, glycated haemoglobin was significantly associated with mortality from CAD after adjustment for several other cardiovascular risk factors.

In the UKPDS, increased baseline haemoglobin A_{1c} concentration was significantly associated with CAD, although not as strongly as other risk factors such as elevated LDL cholesterol concentration (Figure 16).[75] The modifiable risk factors identified included:
- High LDL cholesterol
- Reduced levels of HDL cholesterol
- Systolic blood pressure
- Haemoglobin A_{1c}
- Tobacco smoking.

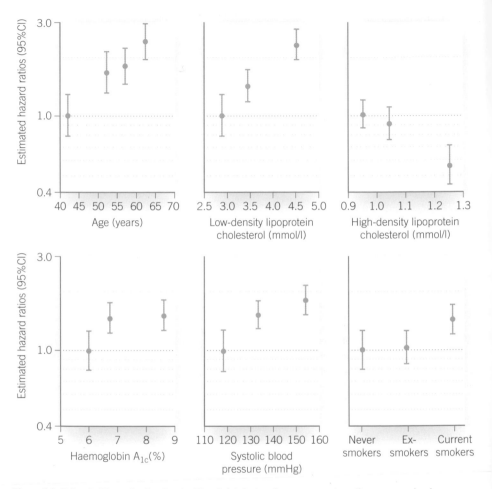

Figure 16. Estimated hazard ratios for significant risk factors for coronary artery disease occurring in 335 out of 3055 patients with diabetes, expressed as floating absolute risks. Reproduced from *BMJ* 1998;316:823–828 with permission from the BMJ Publishing Group.

The results were as follows:

- For each increment of 1 mmol/l in LDL cholesterol concentration there was a 1.57-fold (95% confidence interval 1.37–1.79) increased risk of CAD

- For each positive increment of 0.1 mmol/l in HDL cholesterol concentration there was a 0.15-fold (0.08–0.22) decrease in risk
- For each increment of 10 mmHg in systolic blood pressure there was a 1.15-fold (1.08–1.23) increase in risk
- For each increment of 1% in haemoglobin A_{1c} there was a 1.11-fold (1.02–1.20) increase in risk.

Although it is generally easier to attain control, albeit not perfect, of blood pressure than glycaemia, this is not an excuse for inaction. The interactions between these risk factors are such that clinicians should tackle all of them as effectively as possible.

The level of sustained hyperglycaemia necessary for diagnosing diabetes is based on the risk of long-term microvascular complications, notably retinopathy. However, the glycaemic threshold, which is associated with atherosclerosis, is lower than that for microvascular disease. The term 'dysglycaemia' has been used to bracket together lesser degrees of hyperglycaemia that may nonetheless have implications for CVD.[76] Recent epidemiological data show that the relationship between glycaemia and CVD extends down into the non-diabetic range. Among men in the Norfolk cohort of the European Prospective Investigation into Cancer and Nutrition (EPIC-Norfolk) study, not only did glycated haemoglobin concentration appear to explain most of the excess mortality risk of diabetes, but it also emerged as a continuous risk factor through the whole population distribution;[77] the lowest risk was seen in men with glycated haemoglobin concentrations <5%.

Patients with lesser degrees of glucose intolerance share some of the increased risk of CVD associated with diabetes. This was demonstrated in the Whitehall study of middle-aged male British civil servants using a 50 g oral glucose challenge. CAD mortality was approximately doubled for people with impaired glucose tolerance, defined as a blood glucose above the 95th centile.[78] In a US study that used 1985 WHO diagnostic criteria, a gradient of mortality associated with abnormal glucose tolerance was seen. This ranged from a 40% greater risk in adults with impaired glucose tolerance to a 110% greater risk in adults with clinically evident diabetes (Figure 17). These associations were independent of established CVD risk factors.[79]

More recently, in a report from Finland patients with impaired glucose tolerance diagnosed using 75 g oral glucose tolerance tests, who did not develop diabetes over a 10-year period, were found to be at increased risk of CAD and CVD mortality after adjustments for several potential confounders (Table 9.)[80]

> **"The association between glycaemia and cardiovascular mortality in men extends down into the non-diabetic range"**

Figure 17. Panel A. Cumulative all-cause mortality in 3174 adults aged 30–84 years by glucose tolerance group at baseline. Panel B. Cumulative cardiovascular disease mortality in 3174 adults aged 30–84 years by glucose tolerance group at baseline. (Overall log-rank test p <0.001). Data from the second National Health and Nutrition Survey (NHANES II) in the US. Copyright © 2001 American Diabetes Association. From *Diabetes Care* 2001;24:447–453. Reprinted with permission from *The American Diabetes Association.*

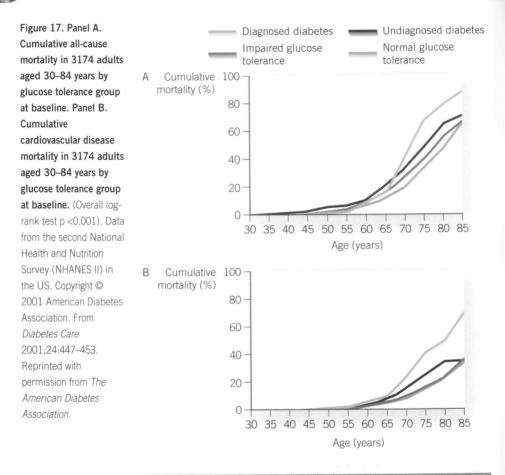

	Hazard ratio	95% Confidence interval
Coronary artery disease incidence	1.49	0.95–2.34
Cardiovascular disease mortality	2.34	1.42–3.85
All-cause mortality	1.65	1.13–2.40

Table 9. Hazard ratios for coronary heart disease incidence, cardiovascular disease mortality and all-cause mortality in subjects with impaired glucose tolerance at baseline who did not go on to develop diabetes. Some 1234 men and 1386 women aged 45–64 years who were free from diabetes at baseline were followed up for 10 years. Copyright © 2003 American Diabetes Association. From Qiao Q *et al. Diabetes Care* 2003;26:2910–2914. Reprinted with permission from *The American Diabetes Association.*

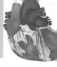

Fasting plasma glucose (mmol/l)	2-Hour plasma glucose (mmol/l)			
	<7.8	7.8–11.0	≥11.1	All categories
<6.1	1.00	1.59 (1.38–1.82)	2.00 (1.46–2.75)	1.00
6.1–6.9	1.19 (1.00–1.42)	1.38 (1.09–1.74)	2.04 (1.35–3.09)	1.20 (1.04–1.38)
7.0–7.7	1.60 (1.04–2.47)	1.59 (1.05–2.41)	2.27 (1.59–3.23)	1.67 (1.32–2.11)
≥7.8	1.41 (0.59–3.42)	1.66 (0.85–3.21)	2.36 (1.80–3.09)	1.94 (1.52–2.47)
All categories	1.00	1.50 (1.33–1.69)	2.13 (1.79–2.52)	

Table 10. Hazard ratios for death (95% confidence intervals) adjusted for age, sex and study centre, according to the fasting glucose and two-hour glucose (post 75 g glucose load) classifications in 18,048 men and 7316 women aged 30 years or older and not known to be diabetic. Reproduced with permission from *Lancet* 1999;354:617 621.

Fasting versus postchallenge hyperglycaemia

As already mentioned, the relationship between impaired fasting glucose and risk of CVD is unclear. In the Diabetes Epidemiology: Collaborative analysis Of Diagnostic criteria in Europe (DECODE) study, baseline data were recorded on fasting and two-hour blood glucose levels in around 18,000 men and around 7300 women aged 30 years or older who had a 75 g oral glucose tolerance test. Mean follow up was seven years. A high blood glucose concentration two hours after the glucose challenge was associated with an increased risk of death, independently of fasting blood glucose. Mortality associated with fasting blood glucose concentration depended on the two-hour blood glucose concentration in all categories of fasting blood glucose (Table 10).[81]

The DECODE study also demonstrated that oral glucose tolerance testing identified more patients with unsuspected diabetes (see above): 31% of 904 patients who were diagnosed as diabetic by glucose tolerance testing had a normal fasting blood glucose, and 20% had impaired fasting glucose. Conversely, among those with diabetes according to the ADA criteria, 59% had two-hour values that failed to meet WHO criteria.

A recent meta-analysis concluded that blood glucose level was a risk marker for CVD even among apparently healthy people without diabetes.[82] Of note, the relative risk of CVD was greater for cohorts that included women (see section on *Diabetes and cardiovascular disease: an intimate relationship*).

The Cardiovascular Health Study has reported that even modest elevations in fasting blood glucose have prognostic implications.[83] Moreover, there is a graded relationship between the extent of vascular disease measured non-invasively and the likelihood of maintaining intact health and function. The implication is that prevention of subclinical vascular disease may increase the quality and the quantity of years in late life.

It does not necessarily follow that elevated postglucose challenge concentrations *per se* are more deleterious than fasting hyperglycaemia.[84] For example, plasma triglycerides also tend to be raised in the presence of glucose intolerance. Therefore, people with IGT have a clustering of classic and non-traditional risk factors for CVD, which may help explain the higher risks associated with elevated two-hour glucose concentrations.[85] Accordingly, it should be noted that, to date, the benefit of selectively targeting postprandial hyperglycaemia using drugs such as the rapid-acting insulin secretagogues repaglinide and nateglinide has not been proven. Prospective randomized studies are in progress, including the Diabetes Reduction Assessment with Ramipril and Rosiglitazone Medication (DREAM) and Nateglinide and Valsartan in Impaired Glucose Tolerance Outcomes Research (NAVIGATOR) studies. Both are using a two-by-two factorial design to assess the additional impact of antihypertensive therapy.

Of interest in this context is the recently reported Study TO Prevent Non-Insulin Dependent Diabetes Mellitus (STOP-NIDDM) trial. In this placebo-controlled randomized study, the alpha-glucosidase inhibitor acarbose, which lowers postprandial hyperglycaemia by slowing intestinal glucose absorption, reduced not only the incidence of new cases of type 2 diabetes in people with impaired glucose tolerance, but also incident cases of MI and new cases of hypertension.[86] An attenuated progression of carotid intima media thickening was also observed.[87] The investigators suggest that reduced oxidative stress, resulting from lowered postprandial glucose levels, may be responsible for their findings.

The common soil hypothesis

In the 1980s, British epidemiologist Professor John Jarrett proposed that the close relationship between hyperglycaemia and atherosclerosis, which he and his colleagues had documented, might reflect shared pathogenic mechanisms (Figure 18). This concept has come to be known as the common soil hypothesis.[88] Of the putative mechanisms linking type 2 diabetes and CVD, the metabolic syndrome (see section below on *Dyslipidaemia*) has been the subject of considerable scrutiny.

Controversially, it has recently been suggested that the risk of microvascular complications, such as retinopathy, neuropathy and nephropathy, may be increased in the presence of degrees of chronic hyperglycemia, i.e. impaired glucose tolerance, that do not satisfy current diagnostic criteria for diabetes mellitus.[89] If confirmed, this would expand the contribution of hyperglycaemia to chronic ill health. Through secondary effects, such as glycation of structural proteins,

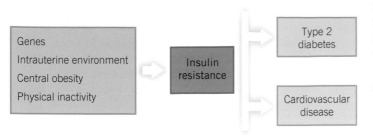

Figure 18. A model of the common soil hypothesis. Adapted from Krentz AJ. *Br J Diabetes Vasc Dis* 2002;2:370–378.

such as collagen, chronic elevations of blood glucose could theoretically contribute to more subtle impairment of functional capacity.[71] Interactions with dietary consumption of fats and impaired renal function may contribute to such an effect.[160]

Dyslipidaemia

The relationship between plasma cholesterol concentration and risk of CVD is similar among patients with diabetes compared with the background population, i.e. there is a curvilinear increase in risk as mean cholesterol concentration rises. However, the risk at any level of cholesterol is higher in the diabetic patient (Figure 7).

“At any given serum cholesterol concentration, the presence of diabetes increases the risk of coronary artery disease by two- to three-fold”

Studies from representative samples of the population of the US show that Asians, Hispanics and American Indians have lower total cholesterol concentrations than non-Hispanic whites. The data also show that these groups have correspondingly lower rates of mortality, with Native Americans and Hispanics also having the lowest stroke rates, even though they have higher rates of type 2 diabetes and insulin resistance. Black people with type 2 diabetes have lower triglyceride and higher levels of HDL cholesterol than their white European counterparts. This may explain the relatively low rates of CAD in people of subSaharan African descent with type 2 diabetes. The discrepancy between the relatively high rates of insulin resistance and lower prevalence of dyslipidaemia and CVD has not been fully explained. In contrast, South Asians tend to have low levels of HDL that are associated with insulin resistance and increased risk of CAD.

Around 35% of adult men and 15% of adult women in the US have HDL cholesterol concentrations less than 1.0 mmol/l. The Münster Heart Study of middle-aged men in Germany demonstrated the risk of a particular lipid profile:

- Reduced levels of HDL cholesterol with a correspondingly high total to HDL ratio
- High triglyceride concentrations
- High concentrations of triglyceride-rich lipoprotein remnants.

Individuals with this 'atherogenic profile' tend to have abdominal obesity and insulin resistance; this is also the profile commonly found in people with type 2 diabetes. There appears to be some overlap with familial combined dyslipidaemia, a common condition responsible for an additional 10–20% of premature CAD.[90] Patients with treated diabetes do not usually have raised absolute levels of total or LDL cholesterol.[91]

"Type 2 diabetes is associated with an atherogenic profile of increased triglyceride and decreased level of HDL cholesterol concentrations"

As discussed later, patients with type 2 diabetes more often have raised levels of fasting and postprandial triglycerides; this is generally accompanied by a low plasma concentration of cardioprotective HDL cholesterol. A high plasma triglyceride concentration is a risk factor for CAD. In multivariate analyses, particularly when correcting for HDL cholesterol, the effect of triglycerides is attenuated, but meta-analysis suggests that triglycerides remain an independent risk factor.[92] Hypertriglyceridaemia is also associated with a high risk of CAD in prospective studies; it has also been shown to be a risk factor for CAD, independent of other lipoprotein concentrations.

Exaggerated postprandial lipaemia is a well-recognized feature of insulin resistance and postprandial hypertriglyceridaemia.[93] In patients with type 2 diabetes, glycaemic control is inversely related to the concentration of postprandial chylomicrons and apolipoprotein B100-containing triglyceride-rich lipoproteins (very-low-density lipoprotein [VLDL] particles and intermediate-density lipoprotein [IDL]). The magnitude and duration of postprandial lipaemia determine the rate of production of atherogenic particles such as small, dense LDL and lipid-depleted HDL, and may also determine clotting system activation, particularly factor VII. Triglyceride-rich remnant particles may be directly related to the development of coronary atheroma.

"The magnitude and duration of postprandial lipaemia determines the rate of production of atherogenic particles such as small, dense LDL and lipid-depleted HDL cholesterol"

Apolipoprotein B48, the main apolipoprotein associated with chylomicrons, can enter the arterial intima and chylomicron remnant concentration correlates with the rate of angiographic progression of coronary disease. Therefore, low triglyceride metabolic capacity, especially in the postprandial period, may be a key feature underlying the development of CAD in insulin-resistant patients.

Low levels of HDL cholesterol are closely associated with increased risk of CAD in both diabetic and non-diabetic populations. There are several reasons for these apparent protective properties of HDL cholesterol. The most obvious is that the main function of HDL is to deliver cholesterol to the liver for excretion. HDL may also have anti-inflammatory and antioxidant properties, protecting against atheromatous disease. The alterations in triglycerides and HDL cholesterol observed among patients with type 2 diabetes tend to be more marked in women than men.[94] This may be part of the explanation for the greater relative risk for women with diabetes.

Other proatherogenic abnormalities associated with type 2 diabetes include the following.

- Small, dense LDL cholesterol – increased levels of small, dense low-density lipoprotein particles (LDL_3), which, it is believed, are more easily oxidized. Oxidized LDL is thought to be toxic to endothelium causing disruption of the endothelium and increased adhesiveness. It may also inactivate nitric oxide, thereby impairing endothelium-dependent vasodilatation. Small, dense LDL particles start to predominate when the serum triglyceride concentration exceeds around 1.5 mmol/l.

- Glycation – the post-translational non-enzymatic modification by hyperglycaemia of lipoproteins, tissue receptors and glycosaminoglycans in the walls of blood vessels, diminishing the ability of apolipoprotein B to act as a ligand for the LDL receptor. Because this is usually the main method by which LDL is removed from the circulation, this results in an increased uptake by scavenger receptors on cells such as macrophages, potentially increasing atheromatous plaque formation.

"Small, dense LDL cholesterol particles have enhanced atherogenicity; glycation may contribute to atherogenesis in patients with diabetes"

Pathogenesis of diabetic dyslipidaemia

In healthy people, circulating insulin efficiently regulates adipocyte lipid metabolism:

- Insulin suppresses intra-adipocyte hormone-sensitive lipase in the postprandial period, preventing lipolysis and resultant release of fatty acids
- Intravascular lipoprotein lipase is stimulated by the higher insulin levels that accompany the early postprandial period; this increases triglyceride clearance from chylomicrons and VLDL particles into adipocytes and, to a lesser extent, into myocytes
- Simultaneously, insulin stimulates intra-adipocyte esterification of fatty acids forming new intra-adipocyte triglyceride stores.

The pattern of dyslipidaemia seen in people with type 2 diabetes is related to insulin resistance and is also apparent in their non-diabetic, insulin-resistant relatives, suggesting that it precedes the development of type 2 diabetes. These processes are impaired as a consequence of defective intracellular insulin signalling. The fatty acids liberated by impaired actions of insulin in adipocytes have been implicated in a diverse range of defects in type 2 diabetes, ranging from hypertriglyceridaemia to impaired insulin secretion and endothelial dysfunction.

Defects typically encountered in type 2 diabetes include:

- Increased hepatic synthesis and secretion of large VLDL particles – this is due, in part, to increased availability of fatty acids. The relationship between this process and the pathogenesis of hepatic

"Increased non-esterified fatty acid concentrations contribute to increased VLDL triglyceride concentrations"

45

steatosis and steatohepatitis (see section on *Diabetes and cardiovascular disease: an intimate relationship*) is uncertain

- Increased residence time of triglyceride-rich particles – particularly as remnant particles, i.e. chylomicron remnants and partially degraded VLDL and IDL particles (Figure 19)
- Increased triglyceride-cholesteryl ester exchange – this occurs between the cholesterol-rich HDL and LDL and the triglyceride-rich VLDL particles and chylomicrons by cholesteryl ester transfer protein (Figure 20)
- Relatively cholesterol-depleted HDL and LDL – these arise as a result of the aforementioned exchanges, together with a reduction in their size due to the hydrolysis of their comparatively triglyceride-rich cores by increased hepatic lipase activity
- Impaired hepatic apolipoprotein A1 production – normally, this unites with phospholipids to form nascent HDL particles. HDL may also be formed by apolipoprotein A1 and phospholipid shed from the surface of VLDL during hydrolysis by lipoprotein lipase. Because lipoprotein lipase activity is decreased in insulin-resistant states, production by this process is also decreased, leading to an overall reduction in synthesis. The major effects of insulin resistance on lipid metabolism are summarized in Table 11.

Figure 19. Elevated portal vein fatty acid levels, arising from insulin resistance in adipocytes, lead to an overproduction of apolipoprotein B-containing particles. Apo B is the structural protein of atherogenic lipoproteins, including very-low-density lipoprotein (VLDL) and intermediate-density lipoprotein (IDL). The apo B concentration reflects the total number of atherogenic particles in the blood. The metabolic syndrome is associated with increased numbers of small VLDL, IDL and low-density lipoprotein (LDL) particles, with a decreased triglyceride (TG) to apo B ratio. (CE = cholesterol ester.) Reproduced with permission from *J Clin Endocrinol Metab* 2004;89:2601–2607.

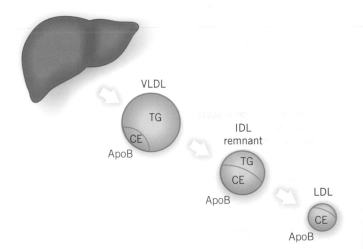

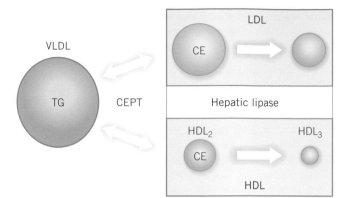

Figure 20. Lipoprotein particle remodelling. Cholesteryl ester transfer protein (CETP) facilitates the exchange of cholesterol ester (CE) in low-density lipoprotein (LDL) and high-density lipoprotein (HDL) particles for triglyceride in very-low-density lipoprotein (VLDL) particles. The transfer of triglyceride (TG) into LDL and HDL particles makes them triglyceride-rich and therefore a better substrate for hepatic lipase. Elevated hepatic lipase activity leads to a predominance of small, dense LDL particles and a reduction in HDL_2, the more antiatherogenic subspecies of HDL. Reproduced with permission from *J Clin Endocrinol Metab* 2004;89:2601–2607.

Decreased suppression of adipocyte hormone sensitive lipase

- Results in continued lipolysis and fatty acid release from adipose tissue in the early postprandial period; this would be suppressed in an insulin-sensitive individual
- Hepatic VLDL production is increased in part due to delivery of fatty acids via the portal vein

Decreased suppression of hepatic VLDL synthesis

- Hepatic production of large VLDL particles is normally suppressed by insulin, but in individuals with insulin resistance there is continued production

Impaired stimulation of lipoprotein lipase

- Clearance of chylomicrons and VLDL is reduced by the relative insensitivity of lipoprotein lipase in muscle and adipose tissue to insulin
- HDL particle formation is decreased due to the decrease in shedding of apolipoprotein A1 and phospholipids from the surface of VLDL during hydrolysis by lipoprotein lipase

Impaired stimulation of intra-adipocyte esterification

- Fatty acid esterification and, therefore, uptake is reduced, further increasing plasma concentrations

VLDL = very-low-density lipoprotein

Table 11. Key effects of insulin resistance on lipid metabolism.

- Increased apolipoprotein B concentration – this is another feature of the dyslipidaemia seen in type 2 diabetes. Apolipoprotein B is necessary for the hepatic secretion of VLDL, there being one apolipoprotein B molecule on each VLDL particle. This is cleared from the circulation (as IDL or LDL). The total concentration of VLDL, IDL and LDL particles is therefore reflected in the apolipoprotein B concentration. In people with type 1 or type 2 diabetes, apolipoprotein B may become glycated, slowing hepatic LDL clearance because of interference with the reaction with the hepatic LDL receptor. Therefore, the plasma half-life of apolipoprotein B is increased. Around 50% of patients with type 2

Figure 21. Odds ratios for coronary artery disease according to plasma insulin and triglyceride concentrations, total:HDL cholesterol ratios, and apolipoprotein B concentrations (HDL = high-density lipoprotein). Reproduced with permission from *N Engl J Med* 1996;334:952–957. Copyright © 1996 Massachusetts Medical Society. All rights reserved.

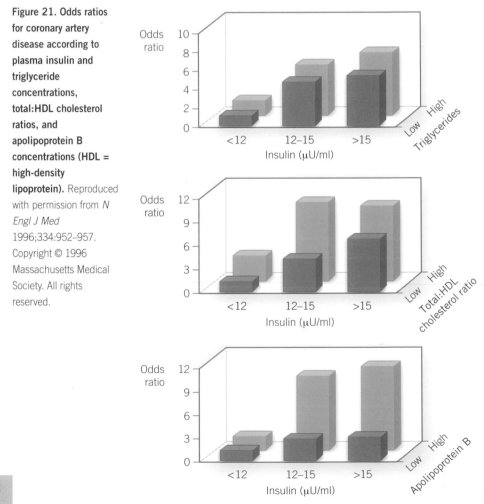

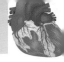

diabetes, who have normal absolute cholesterol levels, have increased apolipoprotein B concentrations. This is often accompanied by the typical pattern of hypertriglyceridaemia and low HDL cholesterol levels. The Quebec Study of non-diabetic middle-aged men showed a striking interaction between high apolipoprotein B and fasting plasma insulin concentrations in predicting coronary events.[95] This serves as an example of the concept that cardiovascular risk may be enhanced by synergistic effects of multiple risk factors (Figure 21).

It has been suggested that increased apolipoprotein B concentrations may be a better predictor of coronary disease in high-risk groups than LDL cholesterol concentrations.[96] However, few centres are currently using apolipoprotein B concentrations routinely in cardiovascular risk calculations.

Currently, guidelines for lipid treatment in people with diabetes are directed at lowering LDL cholesterol, but it is likely that in future more attention will be paid to concentrations other than HDL, particularly in people with the metabolic syndrome. So-called non-HDL cholesterol is an emerging marker of cardiac risk. It is calculated as the difference between total serum cholesterol and HDL cholesterol concentrations. This concept acknowledges the atherogenic potential of all the cholesterol fractions other than HDL cholesterol. In the Strong Heart Study, the highest tertile of non-HDL cholesterol was a better predictor of CVD in American Indian men and women with type 2 diabetes than either LDL cholesterol or triglyceride concentrations.[97]

> *Small, dense LDL cholesterol is more readily oxidized or glycated and is more slowly removed by cellular receptors than large buoyant particles*

Lipids in type 1 diabetes

In patients with treated type 1 diabetes, HDL cholesterol levels may be normal or high, but do not always protect fully against the development of CAD. In patients with severe insulin deficiency, there is a marked acceleration of lipolysis with major derangements of lipid metabolism (Table 12).

This situation is often accompanied by elevated levels of other hormones, for example catecholamines and glucagon, which antagonize the actions of insulin. In the absence of treatment with sufficient exogenous insulin, hepatic ketogenesis develops, fuelled by excessive rates of delivery of fatty acids. This catabolic state may culminate in life-threatening diabetic ketoacidosis. Major states of acute dyslipidaemia, with eruptive xanthomata and lipaemia retinalis reflecting major hypertriglyceridaemia, may occur; these usually resolve promptly with adequate insulin and may reflect co-existing genetic defects in lipid regulation that are exposed by insulin deficiency.

> *Decompensated diabetes may be associated with severe hypertriglyceridaemia*

Table 12. Lipid abnormalities associated with type 1 and type 2 diabetes.

Type 1 diabetes* (related to lack of insulin)	Type 2 diabetes† (related to insulin resistance)
↑ LDL cholesterol	Normal LDL cholesterol But ↑ small, dense LDL cholesterol
↑ Triglyceride	
↑ VLDL synthesis	↑ Triglyceride, particularly postprandially
↓ VLDL and chylomicron clearance	↑ VLDL synthesis
	↓ VLDL and chylomicron clearance
↓ HDL cholesterol	↓ HDL cholesterol

* In well-controlled diabetes, the lipid profile is not usually deranged
† The dyslipidaemia seen in type 2 diabetes is not usually completely reversed by tight metabolic control

"CVD is the major cause of premature mortality in patients with type 2 diabetes, and hypertension is a major contributor to the development of CVD and renal disease in these patients." John R Sowers, 2004[98]

High blood pressure

Hypertension has a major adverse impact on vascular disease and is highly prevalent among patients with type 2 diabetes. Indeed, hypertension, defined as a blood pressure ≥140/90 mmHg, is twice as common among people with diabetes. Overall, around 65% of patients with type 2 diabetes of more than 30 years duration have hypertension, defined as a seated blood pressure >140/90 mmHg. It is thought that high blood pressure accounts for up to 75% of added cardiovascular risk in people with diabetes, contributing significantly to the overall morbidity and mortality.[99] Middle-aged women with diabetes are more likely to have high blood pressure than men.[100]

Among patients with type 2 diabetes, hypertension is often regarded as being an intrinsic facet of the insulin resistance syndrome. However, the mechanistic links between insulin resistance and high blood pressure have not been clearly delineated. The interrelationships between insulin resistance, sympathetic overactivity and activation of the renin-angiotensin system are complex.[101] Recent insights from drug interventions have provided new knowledge of these associations (see section on *Prevention and treatment: current and emerging strategies*).

"Hypertension is around twice as frequent among people with diabetes"

Obesity has a well-recognized effect on blood pressure: mean arterial pressure rises an average of 1 mmHg for every kilogram of body weight. Insulin resistance has been implicated in the pathogenesis of hypertension, although the precise mechanisms are uncertain (Table 13).[102]

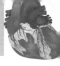

Decreased vascular sensitivity to insulin
• Reduced insulin-induced vasodilatation in capacitance and resistance vessels

Effects of hyperinsulinaemia
• Sodium and water retention due to insulin action on distal renal tubule
• Increased contractility and vascular resistance due to increased systolic calcium concentrations. The latter are secondary to increased vascular smooth muscle intracellular sodium concentrations as a result of insulin stimulation of cell membrane Na+ K+ ATPase.
• Increased sympathetic outflow through effects of insulin within the central nervous system; no direct evidence for this mechanism in humans
• Increased peripheral vascular resistance caused by insulin stimulation of vascular smooth muscle cell proliferation

ATP = adenosine triphosphate

Table 13. Potential mechanisms by which insulin resistance may cause hypertension.

Hypertension is present in around 10–30% of patients with type 1 diabetes, a particularly close association being evident with nephropathy. Blood pressure usually starts to rise in the early stages of diabetic nephropathy, when the albumin excretion rate exceeds 30 mg/24 hours – the somewhat inelegantly named 'microalbuminuria' range. By the time the patient has 'clinical' dipstick-positive proteinuria (albumin excretion rate >300 mg/24 hours) hypertension is usually apparent, and difficult to control. Note that blood pressures <140/90 mmHg may be higher than expected, particularly in younger patients.

Blood pressure tends to rise gradually, although remaining within the non-hypertensive range, as nephropathy progresses. The concept of 'abnormally high blood pressure', irrespective of the presence or absence of diabetes and below the current threshold for diagnosis of hypertension, was enshrined in the seventh report of the Joint National Committee on Prevention, Detection, Evaluation, and Treatment of High Blood Pressure (JNC 7).[103] Therefore, sustained blood pressures of 120–139 mmHg systolic, or 80–90 mmHg diastolic, are now regarded as 'pre-hypertension' (Table 14). For any given level of blood pressure, however, the clinical impact is greater in the presence of diabetes, especially when accompanied by nephropathy.

In healthy people, blood pressure normally has a circadian rhythm with a physiological fall in systolic and diastolic pressures during the night. This nocturnal decline during sleep may be attenuated early in the course of diabetic nephropathy. Therefore, the 24-hour mean blood

"Insulin resistance may be causally implicated in the pathogenesis of hypertension in type 2 diabetes"

"Hypertension is closely associated with nephropathy in patients with diabetes"

BP classification	Systolic BP (mmHg*)		Diastolic BP (mmHg*)	Management*		
					Initial drug therapy	
				Lifestyle modification	Without compelling indication	With compelling indication†
Normal	<120	and	<80	Encourage		
Pre-hypertension	120–139	or	80–89	Yes	No anti-hypertensive drug indicated	Drug(s) for the compelling indications‡
Stage 1 hypertension	140–159	or	90–99	Yes	Thiazide-type diuretics for most: may consider ACE inhibitor, ARB, beta-blocker, CCB or combination	Drug(s) for the compelling indications. Other anti-hypertensive drugs (diuretics, ACE inhibitor, ARB, beta-blocker, CCB) as needed
Stage 2 hypertension	≥160	or	≥100	Yes	Two-drug combination for most (usually thiazide-type diuretic and ACE inhibitor, ARB, beta-blocker or CCB)§	Drug(s) for compelling indications. Other anti-hypertensive drugs (diuretics, ACE inhibitor, ARB, beta-blocker or CCB) as needed

ACE = angiotensin converting enzyme; ARB = angiotensin receptor blocker; BP = blood pressure; CCB = calcium channel blocker
* Treatment determined by highest BP category
† See Table 6
‡ Treat patients with chronic kidney disease or diabetes to BP goal of <130/80 mmHg
§ Initial combined therapy should be used cautiously in those at risk of orthostatic hypotension

Table 14. Classification and management of blood pressure in adults aged 18 years or older according to the seventh report of the Joint National Committee on Prevention, Detection, Evaluation, and Treatment of High Blood Pressure (JNC 7). Reproduced from Chobanian AV et al. JAMA 2003;289:2560–2572.

pressure is elevated. Having said this, the role of 24-hour blood pressure monitoring, which allows the nocturnal decline to be measured, in the diagnosis and management of hypertension has yet to be clearly delineated.

Other pathophysiological mechanisms of hypertension-mediated tissue damage in patients with diabetes include:

- Impaired vascular autoregulation – impaired autoregulation in vulnerable vascular beds, such as those of the retina and renal glomerulus resulting from hyperglycaemia, allows transmission of high systemic blood pressure to the microvasculature

- Decreased vascular compliance – decreased compliance of major vessels, for example the aorta, perhaps resulting from non-enzymatic glycation of vessel wall proteins (see above), may result in higher central pressures. There is a relatively high prevalence of isolated systolic hypertension among middle-aged patients with type 2 diabetes
- Increased blood pressure variability – increased variability of intraindividual blood pressure readings in patients with diabetes has been reported during 24-hour ambulatory recordings
- Endothelial dysfunction – this is a frequent accompaniment of hypertension. Many of the components of the metabolic syndrome, for example dyslipidaemia and chronic inflammation, are associated with impaired endothelial responses as determined by pharmacological challenges under experimental conditions
- Sodium retention – hypertension in patients with type 2 diabetes tends to be characterized by sodium retention and volume expansion, perhaps reflecting effects of hyperinsulinaemia on renal ion handling
- Severe hypoglycaemia – this is a risk of insulin therapy, although sulphonylureas can also cause hypoglycaemia that, in turn, may be associated with acute changes in blood pressure. While sympatho-adrenal activation may have adverse effects on vulnerable vascular beds, the clinical impact of such episodes is uncertain.

A substantial body of evidence is available that strongly supports the use of rigorous therapeutic intervention to reduce elevated blood pressure in patients with diabetes (see section on *Prevention and treatment: current and emerging strategies*). Before initiating treatment, however, a thorough clinical assessment of the diabetic patient with hypertension is required. This should involve the following.

- Exclusion of secondary hypertension – a full medical history and physical examination, and biochemical tests, usually reveal clues about co-existing endocrine causes of hypertension, or other forms of secondary hypertension. However, with the exception of thyroid dysfunction, which is unlikely to present with hypertension, all are uncommon. In the absence of a history of diabetes, or a predisposition because of family history or other major risk factors, endocrine causes of hypertension, for example Cushing's syndrome, acromegaly or phaeochromocytoma, are usually associated with minor degrees of glucose intolerance. However, aggravation of pre-existing diabetes may occur (Table 15).
- Signs of target organ damage including left ventricular hypertrophy, arterial bruits, absent pedal pulses (increased risk of renal

Table 15. Endocrine causes of secondary hypertension. Note that glucose intolerance may be associated directly or indirectly with each of these disorders.

Primary hypothyroidism
Thyrotoxicosis
Acromegaly
Cushing's syndrome
Conn's syndrome
Phaeochromocytoma

artery stenosis; see below), proteinuria and hypertensive retinal changes, should be sought by clinical examination, biochemical tests and non-invasive imaging.

Commonly requested investigations include:

- Urinalysis to identify clinical proteinuria or, if standard dipstick testing is negative, to exclude the presence of microalbuminuria using either semiquantitative dipstick method or early morning urine for laboratory-measured albumin:creatinine ratio (see below)

- Renal function and serum electrolytes – for renal impairment, hypokalaemia (Conn's or Cushing's syndrome, but more frequently due to diuretic therapy) and hyperkalaemia (potassium-sparing drugs, renal impairment, hyporeninaemic hypoaldosteronism associated with diabetic nephropathy and loss of juxtaglomerular cells). Creatinine clearance may be estimated using the Cockcroft–Gault formula (http://www.nephron.com/cgi-bin/CGSI.cgi)

- Resting 12-lead electrocardiogram, seeking evidence of left ventricular hypertrophy – this indicates an adverse prognosis and is a major indication to lower blood pressure when safe and appropriate to do so. This investigation will also readily detect atrial fibrillation, a common dysrhythmia associated with increased risk of stroke and other manifestations of peripheral arterial embolism

- Echocardiography – this is more sensitive for detecting left ventricular hypertrophy and ischaemic changes. Both are fairly common, have prognostic implications and are often sub-clinical

- Ambulatory blood pressure recording – the role of ambulatory blood pressure recording and home measurements by patients in diagnosis and management of hypertension has not been clearly established. Ambulatory measurements may be useful if there is unusual variability in sequential measurements of pressures measured in clinics, hypertension apparently resistant to three or more drugs, symptoms suggesting hypotension (usually on antihypertensive therapy, but beware diabetic autonomic neuropathy) or a suspicion of 'white coat hypertension'. Patients recording their blood

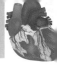

pressure at home should use a validated device, and the reliability of the measurements should be verified if possible

- Other investigations – angiography or isotope studies to exclude clinically significant renal artery stenosis may be indicated in some patients. In general, these investigations are reserved for younger patients with treatment-resistant hypertension. For a patient with characteristic features of progressive diabetic nephropathy, no renal vascular imaging would usually be indicated.

Nephropathy

Diabetes has become the most common single cause of end-stage renal disease in the US and Europe.[104] Renal disease is regarded as a state of accelerated atherosclerosis. Therefore, in both type 1 and type 2 diabetes the development of microalbuminuria heralds an increased risk of CVD. Nephropathy is associated with a clustering of risk factors, including endothelial dysfunction, aspects of which are exacerbated by renal dysfunction.

To put diabetic nephropathy in a broader context, it is becoming increasingly apparent that, in the population at large, relatively minor degrees of renal impairment confer an increased risk of CVD.[105] In particular, a syndrome defined morphologically as focal segmental glomerulosclerosis and glomerulomegaly, known as 'obesity-related glomerulonephropathy', is an increasingly important cause of chronic renal dysfunction.[106] The WHO criteria for the diagnosis of the metabolic syndrome include microalbuminuria as a component (see section on *Diabetes and cardiovascular disease: an intimate relationship*). However, while an association between the metabolic syndrome and chronic renal disease has been reported,[107] this relationship needs further study.

Chronic renal dysfunction has a powerful association with cardiovascular disease

Microalbuminuria

There has been considerable emphasis over the last two decades on the concept of so-called microalbuminuria. This denotes degrees of albuminuria that are higher than normal, but below the level of detection of traditional diagnostic urine sticks, i.e. urinary albumin excretion 30–300 mg daily.

The clinical significance of microalbuminuria derives from its ability to predict progressive renal disease in patients with type 1 and type 2 diabetes. It is also related to premature mortality in patients with diabetes and in the general population. Intervention to preserve glomerular filtration rate and CVD is increasingly being advocated.[108]

A frustrating aspect of diabetic nephropathy is the difficulty of identifying the minority of patients, generally estimated to be around 25–30%, who are at risk of developing it. Genetic analyses are of no value in this regard, or as a guide to treatment. Annual screening for microalbuminuria in patients with diabetes is therefore advocated,[109] although this is fraught with practical and interpretative difficulties. For example, urinary albumin excretion may be transiently increased in the following circumstances:

- Acute metabolic decompensation
- Urinary tract infection
- Heart failure.

Because measurement of 24-hour urinary albumin excretion is obviously not practical, screening test reliance is increasingly being placed on the ratio albumin:creatinine in an early morning urine sample (Figure 22). The upper limits of normal are:

- Men: >2.5 mg/mmol
- Women: >3.5 mg/mmol.

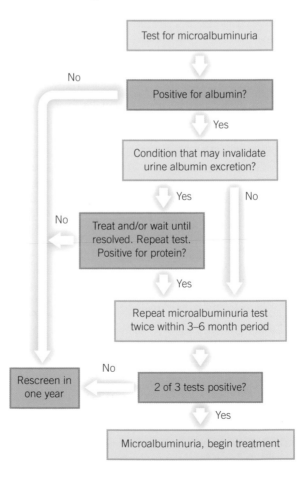

Figure 22. Annual screening for microalbuminuria. The urinary albumin to creatinine ratio is widely recommended for this purpose. Copyright © 2004 American Diabetes Association. From *Diabetes Care* 2004;27:s79–s83. Reprinted with permission from *The American Diabetes Association*.

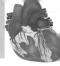

Although patients with microalbuminuria have significant histological renal abnormalities, renal biopsy is not usually needed to diagnose diabetic nephropathy. Microalbuminuria is usually accompanied by a well-preserved glomerular filtration rate. In the absence of therapeutic intervention, progression of nephropathy is the rule; spontaneous regression to normal rates of urinary albumin excretion is rare (see section on *Prevention and treatment: current and emerging strategies*). The presence and magnitude of clinical albuminuria, i.e. >300 mg/day, correlates with loss of renal function.

Clinical assessment should include close monitoring of blood pressure. As nephropathy advances other clinical signs may develop:

- Fluid retention – this may resemble heart failure; indeed, the conditions often co-exist
- Anaemia – this is common and has a multifactorial aetiology; increasingly nephropathy-related anaemia is being managed using recombinant erythropoietin.

Improving glycaemic control, aggressive antihypertensive treatment and the use of ACE inhibitors or angiotensin receptor blockers (ARBs) will slow the rate of progression of nephropathy. In addition, protein restriction and other treatments, such as phosphate lowering, may have benefits in selected patients with more advanced nephropathy. In England and Wales, the National Institute for Clinical Excellence (NICE) recommends early referral for specialist advice for patients with type 2 diabetes, i.e. when the serum creatinine exceeds 150 mmol/l (http://www.nice.org.uk).

66Annual screening of patients with diabetes for microalbuminuria using the urinary albumin to creatinine ratio is widely advocated99

Specialist investigation to exclude alternative causes of renal dysfunction is needed in patients with:

- No microvascular disease in other vascular beds, notably the retina
- Short-duration type 1 diabetes – diabetic nephropathy develops gradually over many years. Note that the difficulty of establishing the onset of type 2 diabetes renders this criterion invalid in these patients
- Rapidly progressive renal dysfunction, i.e. rising serum creatinine, falling glomerular filtration rate
- Nephrotic syndrome – heavy proteinuria with hypoalbuminaemia and peripheral oedema.

The major risk factors for progression from normal urinary albumin excretion to microalbuminuria in patients with diabetes include:

- Levels of albumin excretion approaching the upper limit of normality
- Inadequate long-term glycaemic control
- Elevated blood pressure.

Non-traditional risk factors
The conventional risk factors for CAD include:

- Age
- Elevated serum total cholesterol and LDL cholesterol
- Low levels of HDL cholesterol
- Elevated blood pressure
- Cigarette smoking
- Diabetes
- Vascular disease
- Menopausal status.

The role of so-called novel or non-traditional risk markers is gradually being unravelled (Table 16).[110,111]

A number of non-invasive imaging techniques have also been developed, which have the potential to measure and monitor atherosclerosis in asymptomatic people (Table 17). Some of these, for example coronary calcification scores, may be able to subdivide patients into higher or lesser risk categories within the standard Framingham risk scoring system.

Table 16. Non-traditional risk factors for cardiovascular disease.

- C-reactive protein – a marker of low-grade inflammation
- Fibrinogen – contributes to state of atherothrombosis
- Plasminogen activator inhibitor-1 – impairs fibrinolysis
- Lipoprotein(a) – a plasminogen-like atherogenic molecule
- Homocysteine – high levels associated with atherosclerosis; linked to folate metabolism

Table 17. Non-invasive imaging techniques for assessment of atherosclerosis.

- Exercise electrocardiography
- Ankle-brachial pressure index
- Electron beam computed tomography
- Magnetic resonance coronary angiography
- Positron emission tomography
- B-Mode ultrasound measurement of carotid intima media thickness

C-reactive protein
C-reactive protein is a marker of low-grade systemic inflammation. Increased levels reflect elevated levels of proinflammatory cytokines, notably interleukin-6, which regulates hepatic production of C-reactive protein. Increased levels are associated with insulin resistance, type 2 diabetes and CVD.[112] C-reactive protein can now be measured in serum with highly sensitive assays that measure gradations of the protein within the range previously considered to be normal.

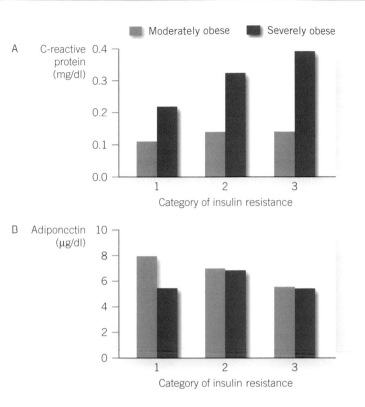

Figure 23. C-reactive protein and adiponectin levels according to the degree of obesity and the insulin-resistance category. Panel A shows C-reactive protein levels (p <0.001 for the association with the obesity group; p = 0.12 for the association with insulin-resistance category; p = 0.64 for the interaction between the obesity group and the insulin-resistance category). Panel B shows adiponectin levels (p = 0.04 for the association with the obesity group; p = 0.005 for the association with the insulin-resistance category; p = 0.07 for the interaction between the obesity group and the insulin-resistance category). After stratification according to the obesity group, the effect of the insulin-resistance category was evident in moderately obese patients; those in the highest category of insulin resistance had significantly lower adiponectin levels than those in the middle and low categories (p = 0.04 and p = 0.002, respectively, with Holm's adjustment). Reproduced with permission from *N Engl J Med* 2004;350: 2362–2374. Copyright © 2004 Massachusetts Medical Society. All rights reserved.

The association of C-reactive protein with CVD has been documented in two large observational studies: the Physicians' Health Study[113] and the Women's Health Study.[114] In the former study, participants in the highest quartile of C-reactive protein at baseline had a higher risk of stroke, MI and severe peripheral arterial disease. The risk associated with high-sensitivity C-reactive protein was independent of other risk factors (Figure 23). Similar results were reported in the Women's Health Study.

In a more recent report in a large cohort of women, C-reactive protein levels increased in line with increasing numbers of components of the metabolic syndrome. At all levels of severity of the metabolic syndrome, however, C-reactive protein added prognostic information on subsequent risk of CVD.[115]

Homocysteine

Elevated serum homocysteine levels have been shown to correlate with risk of CAD in cross-sectional studies, although data are conflicting in prospective studies.[116] Patients with elevated homocysteine levels should be advised to consume the recommended dietary allowance of folic acid.

Whether these markers are causally related to CVD and, if so, to what degree is currently unclear. None of the major coronary heart or cardiovascular risk calculators, for example the Framingham Scoring System, incorporates these novel markers. Some clinicians incorporate them into decision making when considering drug therapy. A family history of premature atherosclerosis is another, perhaps even more important, consideration that is not included in traditional risk factor calculations.

Currently, no data showing that routine testing of patients with diabetes for these risk factors leads to better diagnostic or therapeutic outcomes have been published. What is becoming clear, however, is that improved risk assessment and more sensitive non-invasive imaging are obscuring the traditional line between primary and secondary prevention. The availability and application of these techniques vary markedly between countries.

"The value of using non-traditional risk factors for cardiovascular disease has yet to be determined"

PREVENTION AND TREATMENT: CURRENT AND EMERGING STRATEGIES

Risk factors such as hyperglycaemia, hypertension and dyslipidaemia are amenable to effective therapeutic intervention. However, while non-pharmacological measures are always used as first-line treatment, it is clear that many patients will need adjunctive drug therapy. The widespread use of relatively expensive drugs, such as statins, has obvious implications for primary care clinicians and for increasingly stretched healthcare budgets. Much of the burden of CVD is found in emerging nations who are at a particular disadvantage in this respect.

Furthermore, the increasing prevalence of cardiovascular risk factors among ever younger patients raises concerns of a high toll from CVD in coming years (see section on *Diabetes and cardiovascular disease: an intimate relationship*).[10] Recent studies have illustrated the threat, showing that the prevalence of the metabolic syndrome is high among obese children and adolescents, increasing with greater degrees of obesity. Biomarkers suggesting an increased risk of adverse cardiovascular outcomes, for example reduced adiponectin levels and increased levels of C-reactive protein, are already present in these young people, increasing in line with worsening insulin resistance (Figure 23).[117] Obesity in children is also associated with increased stiffness of the carotid artery, again suggesting higher risk of future cardiovascular events.[118]

There is abundant evidence that control of modifiable risk factors is suboptimal in many patients. Data from the US Third National Health and Nutrition Examination Survey conducted in 1988–1994 and 1999–2000 have recently confirmed this picture with negligible improvement in the intervening years[119]. Only around 7% of adults with diabetes in the 1999–2000 survey attained the recommended goals of haemoglobin A_{1c} level <7%, blood pressure <130/80 mmHg and total cholesterol level <5.18 mmol/l.

> *Since most patients with diabetes die from complications of atherosclerosis, they should receive intensive preventive interventions proven to reduce their cardiovascular risk.* Joshua Beckman *et al*, 2002[1]

Prevention of type 2 diabetes: role of diet, exercise and drugs

There is now good evidence on which to base strategies to prevent type 2 diabetes.[120,121] Two randomized studies, which are supported by other reports, have shown that intensive lifestyle measures, i.e. dietary modification and increased exercise levels, can delay the progression from impaired glucose tolerance to type 2 diabetes in obese patients by 58%. A combination of weight loss and increased exercise levels was most effective; patients reaching their targets had the lowest

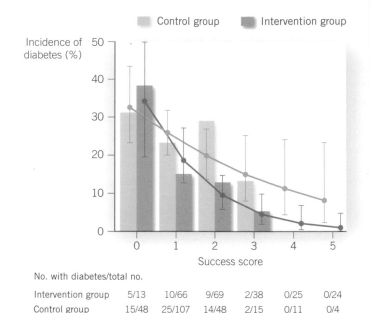

	Intervention group	Control group

No. with diabetes/total no.

Intervention group	5/13	10/66	9/69	2/38	0/25	0/24
Control group	15/48	25/107	14/48	2/15	0/11	0/4

Figure 24. Incidence of diabetes during follow up, according to the success score in the Finnish Diabetes Prevention Study. At the one-year visit, each patient received a grade of 0 for each intervention goal that had not been achieved and a grade of 1 for each goal that had been achieved; the success score was calculated as the sum of the grades. Forty patients who withdrew from the study when their diabetes status was unknown and 14 patients with incomplete data were excluded from this analysis. The association between the success score and the risk of diabetes, with 95% confidence intervals, was estimated by logistic-regression analysis of the observed data. The curves show the model-based incidence of diabetes according to the success score as a continuous variable; the curve whose data points align with the open bars represents the model-based incidence for the control group, and the curve whose data points align with the shaded bars represents the model-based incidence for the intervention group. The mean body mass index at entry was 34 kg/m^2. Reproduced with permission from *N Engl J Med* 2001;344:1343–1350. Copyright © 2001 Massachusetts Medical Society. All rights reserved.

risk of progression (Figure 24). Note that physical activity also has an important protective effect against CAD – a fact that is perhaps underappreciated.[122]

A range of chronic diseases, including diabetes and CAD, can be attenuated by 30 minutes or more of moderately intense aerobic activity such as brisk walking or cycling on five or more occasions per week.

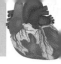

In addition to improvements in blood pressure, lipids profile, insulin sensitivity and body weight, physical activity may improve endothelial function and coronary blood flow, and reduce levels of inflammatory markers and thrombotic risk. Regular exercise also has an important role in cardiac rehabilitation after MI and in the treatment of intermittent claudication.

One of the aforementioned studies, the Diabetes Prevention Program (DPP), also showed that metformin could reduce progression to diabetes by 31% – the drug being more effective in younger patients. Troglitazone was also effective, but this arm of the study was terminated when the drug was withdrawal from the market. The severe idiopathic hepatotoxicity seen with troglitazone is not shared by pioglitazone or rosiglitazone. No drugs are currently licensed for the prevention of type 2 diabetes. As discussed earlier, the increasing global prevalence of diabetes demands effective prevention strategies that are applicable to entire populations, many with limited resources.

> *Delay of progression from impaired glucose tolerance to type 2 diabetes is achievable with intensive lifestyle interventions*

Obesity

As discussed earlier, obesity is a major correlate of type 2 diabetes and an important cause of acquired insulin resistance. Moreover, obesity exacerbates many classic and non-traditional risk factors for CVD. It is fair to say that despite the well-recognized benefits of weight loss on glycaemia, lipids, blood pressure, inflammatory markers and other risk factors, treatment generally remains far from satisfactory. Macronutrient content may independently influence CVD risk factors.

Low-carbohydrate diets

Although low-carbohydrate diets are currently very popular,[123] no randomized trials of more than 12 months' duration have been published. Reductions in triglycerides and elevations in HDL may be offset by increases in LDL concentrations. Limited data suggest that the quality of the LDL is improved, i.e. moving away from the small dense pattern A to the larger buoyant pattern B; the latter is regarded as being less atherogenic. It is unclear whether the changes in lipids are sustained during weight maintenance. Further research is needed before these diets can be recommended for long-term use.

Antiobesity drugs

Studies evaluating the long-term efficacy of antiobesity drugs are currently limited to orlistat and sibutramine. Orlistat is an intestinal lipase inhibitor, whereas sibutramine is a centrally acting serotonin-noradrenaline reuptake inhibitor and an appetite suppressant. Both drugs appear modestly effective in promoting weight loss. Elevations of blood pressure and heart rate may preclude treatment with sibutramine in many patients with diabetes.

A recent Cochrane database systematic review examined the effect of antiobesity drugs.[124] In studies where patients initially received lifestyle modification, compared with placebo patients on orlistat lost 2.7 kg (2.9% less weight) and patients on sibutramine lost 4.3 kg (4.6% less weight). The number of patients achieving ≥10% weight loss was 12% higher with orlistat, and 15% higher with sibutramine. Evaluation of efficacy was, however, limited by high-attrition rates in the studies. The authors concluded that longer and more rigorous studies of antiobesity drugs are needed to examine end points such as mortality and cardiovascular morbidity. In a study of obese patients with normal or impaired glucose tolerance, orlistat reduced the incidence of type 2 diabetes in the latter group, compared with lifestyle changes alone.[125]

Bariatric surgery, in its various forms, is generally more effective than drugs; indeed, it can be very successful at countering cardiovascular risk factors.[126] However, the availability of this treatment is very limited in some countries, the UK being a notable example.

Interest is currently being generated by a new class of agents – the cannabinoid receptors antagonists.[127] Data from clinical studies in men of the first cannabinoid receptor$_1$ antagonist, rimonabant, show:

- Weight loss of several kilograms in those compliant with 20 mg daily
- Reductions in waist circumference
- Improved lipid profiles
- Reduced levels of inflammatory markers
- Improved glucose metabolism and reduced serum insulin levels.

Increases in circulating adiponectin levels (see section on Diabetes and cardiovascular disease: an intimate relationship) may be relevant to some of these changes, such as improvements in HDL. To date, tolerability of rimonabant appears to be good. Long-term safety and efficacy data are needed. Theoretical concerns about pharmacological modulation of brain cannabinoid receptors need careful evaluation.

Certain commonly used drugs may promote or exacerbate obesity:

- Corticosteroids – these drugs have potent weight-promoting actions, particularly at higher doses. The characteristic alteration of body composition is accompanied by insulin resistance
- Psychotropic drugs – many of these agents are associated with weight gain. Much interest has focused recently on the so-called atypical antipsychotics, such as clozapine and olanzapine. Because of the risks of excessive weight gain and the development of the metabolic syndrome these drugs need careful monitoring
- β-blockers – the place of these drugs in the treatment of hypertension

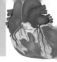

has been questioned, in part because of the potential for weight gain (see below)

- Antiretroviral agents – nucleoside reverse-transcriptase inhibitors, such as stavudine and zidovudine, promote central adiposity and subcutaneous lipoatrophy (see section on *Diabetes and cardiovascular disease: an intimate relationship*)
- Thiazolidinediones – these drugs reduce insulin resistance while promoting weight gain. It is hypothesized that stimulation of subcutaneous adipogenesis redistributes lipid away from the aforementioned ectopic sites (see below)
- Hormonal contraceptive preparations – there is little in the way of hard evidence for an adverse effect of combined oral contraceptives or depot-medroxyprogesterone acetate.

Hyperglycaemia

During the last three decades, major trials have tested the hypothesis that vascular complications of diabetes are determined by the degree and duration of hyperglycaemia. In each study, selected patients were randomly allocated to standard or more intensive therapy, the latter resulting in a sustained improvement in glycaemic control. The Diabetes Control and Complications Trial (DCCT)[128] in patients with type 1 diabetes and the UKPDS[129] in type 2 diabetes demonstrated the importance of long-term glycaemic control in preventing the development and retarding the progression of microvascular tissue complications, i.e. retinopathy, nephropathy and neuropathy.

> **"Major trials have demonstrated the importance of long-term glycaemic control for preventing microvascular complications"**

However, the picture is less clear for macrovascular disease; both of these landmark studies provided equivocal evidence for the importance of treating hyperglycaemia. In part, this dichotomy may reflect the lower glycaemic threshold for risk of atherosclerosis. Therefore, exceptionally good glycaemic control with plasma glucose concentrations consistently in the normal range would be needed. Neither study was able to provide this degree of control – a failure that reflects the inadequacies of antidiabetic drugs, including insulin. In the DCCT, intensified insulin therapy was associated with greater weight gain and a three-fold increase in episodes of severe hypoglycaemia.

Type 1 diabetes

Among the young and relatively healthy patients in the DCCT, a non-significant reduction in macrovascular events was observed in those randomized to intensified insulin therapy. The trial was neither designed nor powered to demonstrate the impact of intensified therapy on macrovascular disease. In a follow-up study, however, carotid intima media thickness, a predictor of macrovascular disease, progressed less rapidly in the intensive treatment group.[130] It seems that a 'legacy effect' of earlier improvements in metabolic control provided continued protection for the macrovasculature.

More persuasive evidence for benefits of near-normalization of blood glucose on macrovascular disease comes from successful pancreatic grafting;[131] carotid intima media thickness improved after pancreas transplantation in the absence of changes in non-glucose cardiovascular risk factors. Data from an observational study showing improved survival among patients with type 1 diabetes and impaired autonomic cardiovascular reflexes, who received a functioning pancreatic transplant, are of interest in this regard.[132]

Type 2 diabetes: oral antidiabetic agents

The treatment of type 2 diabetes conventionally follows a stepwise approach with oral agents being added to lifestyle measures in most patients. All the available classes of orally active drugs have cardiovascular implications; some apparently have benefits, whereas with others there are doubts about safety in high-risk patients (Table 18).

Table 18. Classes of oral antidiabetic agents used to treat type 2 diabetes. Note that availability and preparations differ between countries.

Sulphonylureas
• First generation, e.g. tolbutamide, chlorpropamide • Second generation, e.g. glibenclamide, glipizide, gliclazide, glimepiride
Rapid-acting insulin secretagogues
• Repaglinide • Nateglinide
Biguanides
• Metformin • (Phenformin withdrawn in US and UK in 1977 due to unacceptable risk of lactic acidosis)
Alpha-glucosidase inhibitors

• Acarbose
• Miglitol
• Thiazolidinediones:
   – Rosiglitazone
   – Pioglitazone
   – (Troglitazone withdrawn in 2000 in the US and elsewhere due to idiopathic severe hepatotoxicity)

Sulphonylureas

The seeds of the sulphonylurea controversy were sown in the US in the 1960s. The University Group Diabetes Program (UGDP) made what seemed a laudable, if ultimately flawed, attempt to determine which treatment for diabetes was most efficacious. Briefly, patients with what would now be classified as type 2 diabetes were assigned to different antidiabetic therapies, including insulin, for 3–8 years. The results suggested that improved glucose control by any method did not reduce the risk of cardiovascular end points. Moreover, cardiovascular mortality appeared to be increased in patients treated with a fixed dose of the sulphonylurea tolbutamide.

Much criticism was subsequently heaped on the UGDP for perceived failings in randomization and analysis, which undermined its conclusions.[133] Having said this, the issue of the cardiovascular safety of the sulphonylureas has shown remarkable resilience over the years.

Residual concerns about cardiovascular safety of the sulphonylureas were propagated by the discovery that cardiac muscle and vascular smooth muscle express isoforms of the sulphonylurea receptors SUR2A and SUR2B. Sulphonylureas that contain a benzamido group (glibenclamide, glipizide and glimepiride) can bind to SUR2A/B, whereas those without (such as tolbutamide, chlorpropamide and gliclazide) show very little interaction with the cardiac and vascular sulphonylurea receptors. The effects of the K_{ATP} channel opener nicorandil – an antianginal drug with cardioprotective properties – are blocked by sulphonylureas that have a benzamido group.[134]

The clinical implications of these observations remain to be determined. Very high concentrations of sulphonylureas can cause contraction of cardiac and vascular muscle. Although this is unlikely to be clinically significant at therapeutic drug concentrations, the fixed high dose of tolbutamide used in the UGDP would have maximized the chances of revealing adverse cardiovascular effects.

Other reports continue to foster a vague sense of unease among some clinicians. For example, there is some evidence that sulphonylureas may attenuate the rise in ST segments on the electrocardiogram, an effect with obvious clinical implications.[135] Perhaps understandably, some investigators continue to advocate that use of sulphonylureas be kept to a minimum in patients with overt CAD. In this complex debate, it might be seen as reassuring that the recently reported Steno-2 study[136] showed that macrovascular events, including coronary events, were reduced in high-risk patients with type 2 diabetes using gliclazide as part of a multifactorial approach to therapy (see below). Until this issue is resolved, avoiding sulphonylureas known to have adverse effects on ischaemic preconditioning is an option for patients at high risk of coronary events.

> *Controversy has surrounded the relationship between sulphonylureas and cardiovascular disease for decades*

> *Avoiding sulphonylureas with adverse effects on ischaemic preconditioning may be prudent in patients with type 2 diabetes who have coronary artery disease*

The UKPDS[129] was conceived in the midst of the uncertainty generated by the UGDP. In this 20-year study, 3867 newly diagnosed middle-aged patients with type 2 diabetes were randomized to either an intensive control group aiming for a fasting blood glucose <6 mmol/l or to a less intensive treatment group aiming only for patients to be asymptomatic with a fasting plasma glucose <15 mmol/l. In the intensive treatment group, patients were primarily treated with either a sulphonylurea or, in contrast to usual UK clinical practice, insulin.

During the 10-year follow up, the median HbA_{1c} was 0.9% lower (7.0% versus 7.9%) in the intensively treated group. Although this reduced microvascular complications, the reduction in MI was not statistically significant (relative risk 0.84; 95% confidence interval 0.7–1.0; p = 0.052).[129] Reassuringly, however, there was no evidence of increased mortality in patients randomized to sulphonylurea treatment. The reasons for the borderline statistical significance may, in part, reflect the exclusion of many patients at highest risk, i.e. those with clinically evident atherosclerosis, which reduced the power of the study.

A subsequent observational analysis (UKPDS 35) of data for the entire cohort, i.e. combining the intensive and conventional treatment groups, indicated that for each 1% reduction in glycated haemoglobin there was a 14% reduction in MI (95% confidence interval 8–21%; p<0.0001) and a 21% reduction for deaths related to diabetes (15–27%; p <0.0001).[137] In Figure 25, the slope of the regression line for the relationship between hazard ratio and updated mean haemoglobin A_{1c} is less steep for fatal and non-fatal MI than for microvascular end points, explaining the greater benefits observed in the UKPDS on microvascular events with improved glycaemic control.

Since the conclusion of the randomized phase of the UKPDS, when allocation to intensive and conventional treatment groups was no longer maintained, reanalysis with a longer period of follow up showed that the difference in MI rates between the groups achieved statistical significance. This occurred despite some convergence between the original groups in terms of glycaemic control. A degree of caution is perhaps appropriate, however, in view of the multiple statistical analyses of these data.

Rapid-acting insulin secretagogues
There are currently no clinical outcome data for repaglinide or nateglinide with respect to vascular events.

Metformin
Of note in the UKPDS, only patients randomized to receive metformin as monotherapy had a decreased mortality from MI;[75] these

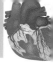

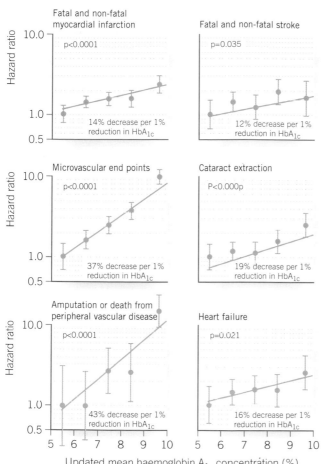

Figure 25. Hazard ratios, with 95% confidence intervals as floating absolute risks, as an estimate of association between category of updated mean haemoglobin A_{1c} concentration and myocardial infarction, stroke, microvascular end points, cataract extraction, lower extremity amputation or fatal peripheral vascular disease and heart failure. Reference category (hazard ratio 1.0) is haemoglobin A_{1c} <6% with log linear scales. p value reflects contribution of glycaemia to multivariate model. Data adjusted for age at diagnosis of diabetes, sex, ethnic group, smoking, presence of albuminuria, systolic blood pressure, high-density lipoprotein and low-density lipoprotein cholesterol and triglycerides. Reproduced from *BMJ* 2000;321:405–412 with permission from the BMJ Publishing Group.

patients also had a significantly reduced risk of a diabetes-related death (Table 19). Metformin is not superior to other treatments in improving glycaemic control, but has the advantage of avoiding hyperinsulinaemia. Other putative cardioprotective effects of metformin include reductions in circulating levels of plasminogen activator inhibitor-1. It is also associated with less weight gain than sulphonylureas or insulin.

In obese patients, metformin is widely regarded as the first-line drug of choice, although evidence against benefit was seen in a sub-study of sulphonylurea-treated patients assigned to receive metformin

Table 19. Summary of main results of UKPDS 34: relative reductions in risk with metformin versus conventional (diet) therapy in overweight patients with type 2 diabetes. Data from UKPDS 34: UK Prospective Diabetes Study (UKPDS) Group. Effect of intensive blood-glucose control with metformin on complications in overweight patients with type 2 diabetes. *Lancet* 1998;352:854–865.

	Relative risk for metformin therapy	CI	Log-rank p
Aggregate end points			
Diabetes-related end points	0.68	(0.53–0.87)	0.002
Diabetes-related deaths	0.58	(0.37–0.91)	0.017
All-cause mortality	0.64	(0.45–0.91)	0.011
CI = 95% confidence interval versus conventional (diet) therapy			

therapy because of inadequate glycaemic control.[138] Although this finding caused alarm among UK general practitioners, it has been suggested that it was probably a spurious result. However, a population-based observational study found similar results.[139] In the absence of additional definitive randomized trials, this represents another aspect of the sulphonylurea-CVD controversy.

Use of metformin is often limited by problems with gastrointestinal tolerability. The drug should be avoided in situations where:

*   The drug may accumulate
*   Anaerobic metabolism may be accelerated, for example in patients with cardiac failure.

Renal impairment heads the list of contraindications to metformin because of the risk, albeit small, of lactic acidosis associated with impaired excretion of the drug.[140] Some clinicians take the view that metformin should generally be avoided in patients at high risk of vascular events that, by their nature, may lead to sudden and unpredictable tissue hypoxia. However, some investigators argue that the metabolic and vascular protective effects of metformin might be beneficial in such situations.[141] This controversial view has not been substantiated. At the present time, we continue to advocate a cautious approach.

> **"Use of metformin reduces the risk of cardiovascular disease in overweight patients with type 2 diabetes"**

Thiazolidinediones

Since the results of the UKPDS were published, the thiazolidinediones have been licensed.[142] The currently available drugs, pioglitazone and rosiglitazone, can be used in the UK as monotherapy in selected patients, or in combination with metformin or a sulphonylurea. Thiazolidinediones improve whole-body insulin sensitivity (see section on *Hyperglycaemia*) via multiple actions on gene regulation. These

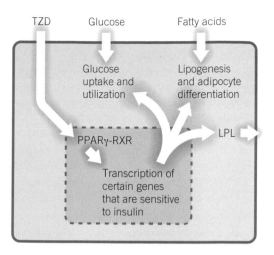

Figure 26. Cellular mechanism of action of thiazolidinediones (TZD) via the peroxisome proliferator-activated receptor gamma retinoid X receptor (PPARγ-RXR), causing transcription of insulin-sensitive genes involved in glucose uptake and lipogenesis. (LPL = lipoprotein lipase). Reproduced from Day C. *Diabetic Med* 1999;16:179–192 with permission from Blackwell Publishing.

effects result from stimulation of a nuclear receptor – peroxisome proliferator-activated receptor-γ (PPAR-γ) – for which thiazolidinediones are potent synthetic agonists (Figure 26).

Binding with the retinoid X receptor forms a heterodimer that acts on response elements on deoxyribonucleic acid. Multiple genes are activated or suppressed in the presence of relevant cofactors.[143] In the presence of sufficient insulin concentrations – like other oral agents they are ineffective in type 1 diabetes – thiazolidinediones reduce circulating levels of glucose and fatty acids. Plasma insulin concentrations decline and measures of islet β-cell function improve.

Evidence from small studies has suggested that these drugs may have beneficial effects beyond glucose lowering.[144] Both drugs have complex effects on dyslipidaemia, including increases in HDL cholesterol levels. Triglyceride levels tend to fall with pioglitazone. Levels of LDL cholesterol may rise with rosiglitazone, although levels of apolipoprotein B decline; the implications of these changes, which could be seen as a combination of potentially advantageous and possible deleterious effects, are unclear at present.[145]

Other potentially anti-atheromatous effects include reduced levels of inflammatory markers such as C-reactive protein (see section on *Cardiovascular risk factors in the patient with diabetes*), lowered levels of plasminogen activator inhbitor-1, and decreases in blood pressure and microalbuminuria. In addition, these drugs may modify pivotal cellular steps in atherogenesis within the arterial wall. Whether such effects will result in a reduction in long-term risk of CVD is unknown; the results of long-term outcome studies with cardiovascular end points are awaited. These include the Prospective Pioglitazone Clinical Trial in

Macrovascular Events (PROactive), the Rosiglitazone Evaluated for Cardiac Outcomes and Regulation of glycaemia in Diabetes (RECORD) and the Bypass Angioplasty Revascularization Investigation in type 2 Diabetes (BARI 2D) trials. The BARI 2D study aims to test the hypothesis that insulin-sensitizing drugs are superior to glycaemic control attained using exogenous insulin or stimulation of exogenous insulin.

To date, studies of surrogate markers of CVD have shown decreased progression of carotid intima media thickness and improvements in endothelial function with thiazolidinediones. In women with PCOS, thiazolidinediones attenuate hyperandrogenism (see section on *Diabetes and cardiovascular disease: an intimate relationship*); ovulation may recommence. These drugs have been linked with intrauterine growth retardation,[145] making them an unattractive treatment for infertility.

> **Thiazolidine-diones may have beneficial cardiovascular effects beyond glucose lowering; the results of outcome trials are awaited**

Unwanted effects of thiazolidinediones include weight gain, averaging 2–4 kg in clinical trials, and peripheral oedema. There have been concerns about precipitating cardiac failure, particularly in patients treated with insulin who seem particularly vulnerable.[146] So-called dual PPAR agonists, which seek to combine the effects of activating PPAR-α and PPAR-γ, are under development. The PPAR-γ is the target for the lipid-modulating fibric acid derivatives, and so it is hoped that advantageous effects of lipid profiles will be seen. However, issues relating to safety or tolerability have led to the curtailment of several promising drugs.

Acarbose

Confirmation of the intriguing findings of the previously discussed STOP-NIDDM trial are awaited. Currently, acarbose is used little in the UK for treating type 2 diabetes, gastrointestinal side effects being a major limiting factor. Enthusiasm has been greater in other countries, such as Germany.

Hyperglycaemia and outcomes after acute MI

> **Hyperglycaemia is associated with worse outcomes in patients with a myocardial infarction**

Short-term hyperglycaemia at the time of an MI, whether or not a patient is known to have diabetes, is associated with increased mortality. In a systematic review patients without diabetes who had glucose concentrations ≥6.1–8.0 mmol/l had a 3.9-fold (95% confidence interval 2.9–5.4) higher risk of death than those without diabetes who had lower glucose concentrations.[147] There is also an association between long-term antecedent glycaemic control and risk of death after MI or stroke. It is now routine practice to measure blood glucose in patients admitted to hospital with acute coronary syndromes, i.e. acute MI or unstable angina.[148]

The high prevalence of clinically significant glucose intolerance among 181 consecutive patients with a mean age of 64 years hospitalized with acute MI was highlighted by a study from Sweden. When patients known to have diabetes were excluded, glucose intolerance or diabetes mellitus was detected in around 60% of the sample. Moreover, fewer than 35% of patients had normal glucose tolerance at repeat assessment using 75 g oral glucose tolerance tests three months later, at which point the effects of MI, left ventricular dysfunction and inflammatory processes should have subsided.[149]

Controlling hyperglycaemia immediately after acute MI using insulin may improve long-term outcome. In another Swedish study, the Diabetes Mellitus and Insulin–Glucose Infusion in Acute Myocardial Infarction (DIGAMI) trial, 620 patients admitted with an MI with blood glucose >11 mmol/l, whether or not they were known to have diabetes, were randomized to receive standard care or to receive an insulin–dextrose infusion, and subsequently to continue insulin for at least three months.[150]

The objective was to control blood glucose concentrations, both during the acute phase of the MI and after discharge from hospital. The use of thrombolytic therapy and other cardioprotective drugs was similar between the groups. At a mean follow up of 3.4 years, there was a significantly lower mortality in the group assigned to intensive treatment (Figure 27).

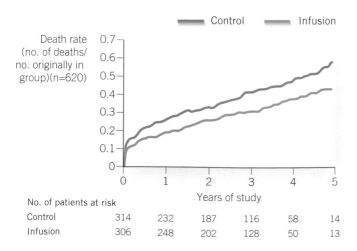

Figure 27. Actuarial mortality curves during long-term follow up in patients receiving insulin-glucose infusion and in a control group among the total DIGAMI cohort (absolute reduction in risk 11%; relative risk 0.72 [0.55–0.92]; p = 0.011). Reproduced from *BMJ* 1997;314:1512–1515 with permission from the BMJ Publishing Group.

The absolute reduction in mortality was 11%, implying one saved life for nine patients treated according to the DIGAMI protocol. Of note, the reduction in risk was largely confined to those patients (n = 272) perceived to be at lowest risk based on pre-specified criteria:

- Age <70 years
- No history of MI or heart failure
- No treatment with digitalis
- Not taking insulin on admission.

Critics were quick to point out that, for several reasons, only half of patients who were eligible on the grounds of blood glucose levels were entered into the study, there was a sizeable drop-out rate from the insulin treatment arm, and a number of patients in the non-intensive arm were transferred to insulin therapy (drop-ins). It was also unclear whether short-term metabolic correction at the time of the MI, or long-term insulin therapy with potentially improved control, was the most important factor. Unfortunately, the follow-up study, DIGAMI 2, which was intended to address these questions, was beset by other methodological problems.

DIGAMI 2 included a total of 1253 patients with suspected acute MI. Patients were randomized to one of three groups:

1. Acute insulin–dextrose infusion followed by insulin-based long-term glucose control
2. Insulin–glucose infusion followed by standard glucose control (i.e. no insulin)
3. Routine metabolic management according to local practice.

The patients in DIGAMI 2 proved to be younger and healthier with a lower mortality rate than anticipated; recruitment was slower than expected leading to early termination of the study. It is possible that recent improvements in coronary care made it more difficult to demonstrate the independent impact of metabolic control. There was no significant difference in mortality between the groups, perhaps partly reflecting protocol lapses. Nevertheless, blood glucose remained an independent predictor of mortality.[151] It seems appropriate to start insulin–dextrose infusion with the aim of controlling hyperglycaemia; subsequent use of insulin after discharge from hospital may be advantageous if it can be safely implemented.

There are sound theoretical reasons why provision of insulin might be beneficial in the setting of acute MI. Myocardial energy production in patients with diabetes is shifted away from glucose oxidation to fatty acid oxidation; this shift generates less adenosine triphosphate per mole of oxygen consumed. This imbalance may be particularly evident within the infarct, wherein the opportunity to create energy is negligible in the diabetic patient. Much of the non-infarcted zone involved in

"An insulin–dextrose infusion followed by subcutaneous insulin may improve long-term outcomes in patients with diabetes after acute MI"

the remodelling process is adversely affected by autonomic neuropathy that contributes to diastolic and systolic dysfunction. Studies of glucose–insulin infusions in non-diabetic patients with acute MI support the protective effects of this approach.[152]

Insulin resistance has been reported in the myocardium of patients with type 2 diabetes;[153] theoretically, this may have implications for insulin doses needed to improve glucose metabolism during myocardial ischaemia. Much more speculative is that the use of insulin brings benefit by eliminating cardiotoxic effects of sulphonylureas, as discussed earlier.

Dyslipidaemia

A recent review of the literature concluded that lipid-lowering in patients with type 2 diabetes reduces cardiovascular risk. This included patients with baseline LDL cholesterol concentrations <3 mmol/l.[154] This view is based on clinical trials that have studied management of hyperlipidaemia in primary and secondary prevention of CVD. Most of the evidence favouring lipid-lowering relates to the use of hydroxy-methyl glutamyl coenzyme A reductase inhibitors – statins; however, there is increasing evidence to suggest benefits from fibrate therapy.

"LDL cholesterol is a poison accentuated by other risk factors"
W Virgil Brown, 2004

The impact of statins has been such that recent trials have been terminated early because pre-specified criteria have been met. This has had the effect of constraining the apparent benefits which may increase with longer duration of treatment. Ethically, however, continued assignment to placebo when benefits are being observed with active treatment is no longer permissible.

Non-pharmacological approaches to treatment

With the increasing evidence of the effectiveness of statins, more and more patients will be treated, but it is still important to remember non-pharmacological measures.

- Dietary measures – attaining ideal body weight, reducing saturated fat consumption to around 30% of total calories, increasing intake of monounsaturates, avoiding *trans*-fatty acids. Excessive alcohol consumption may exacerbate hypertriglyceridaemia. The UKPDS[155] showed that three months' diet therapy (hypocaloric for overweight patients, total maximum fat intake 35% by substitution of polyunsaturated for saturated fats) in newly diagnosed middle-aged patients resulted in a reduction in mean plasma triglycerides (17% in men, 10% in women) with marginal improvements in total cholesterol and cholesterol subfractions. Body weight was reduced by a mean of 5% and fasting plasma glucose was reduced.
- Aerobic physical exercise – this can be useful for reducing

hypertriglyceridaemia and raising HDL cholesterol levels.

- Optimizing diabetic control – hepatic LDL receptors are regulated by insulin; therefore, total and LDL cholesterol levels may decline when hyperglycaemia is adequately treated. Grossly elevated triglyceride levels may respond dramatically to insulin therapy, in conjunction with a low-fat diet. Therefore, changing from oral antidiabetic agents to insulin may help control two major metabolic abnormalities of diabetes. These benefits are logical consequences of countering deficiency of insulin or cellular insulin action.

- Avoiding drugs that exacerbate dyslipidaemia – this includes non-selective ß-blockers and higher doses of thiazide diuretics. However, clinical indications, for example angina pectoris or post-MI, should take precedence over concerns about lipids. The UKPDS found no consistent trends in lipid levels between atenolol- and captopril-based treatments in patients with type 2 diabetes (see below).[156] Other drugs, such as corticosteroids, exacerbate dyslipidaemia as well as hyperglycaemia. Combined oral contraceptives may elevate VLDL triglycerides.[157] However, low-dose oestrogen replacement therapy tends to improve aspects of plasma lipid profiles in postmenopausal women (see section on *Diabetes and cardiovascular disease: an intimate relationship*).

"Always consider causes of secondary hyperlipidaemia "

- Excluding other aggravating factors – hepatic dysfunction, renal impairment and hypothyroidism may cause or exacerbate dyslipidaemia as may certain drugs.

Statins

The Scandinavian Simvastatin Survival Study (4S)[158] and the Cholesterol and Recurrent Events (CARE) trial[159] both included subgroups of patients with diabetes.

The 4S trial

The 4S[158] included 202 patients with diabetes and a previous MI or angina, plasma cholesterol of 5.5–8 mmol/l and triglycerides <2.5 mmol/l. Treatment with simvastatin for a mean of 5.4 years resulted in a reduction in total cholesterol concentrations of 27%, a fall in LDL cholesterol of 36% and in triglycerides of 11%, and an increase in HDL cholesterol of 8%. The relative risk for major CAD events was 0.45 (95% confidence interval 0.27–0.74; p = 0.002), and 0.63 (95% confidence interval 0.43–0.92; p = 0.018) for any atherosclerotic event in the simvastatin-treated patients compared with placebo. Similar results were found in an extended analysis involving a larger proportion of the initial patient cohort, wherein 1997 ADA criteria were used to diagnose diabetes and impaired fasting glucose (i.e. fasting venous plasma glucose concentration >7.0 mmol/l and 6.1–6.9 mmol/l, respectively).[160]

CARE

CARE[159] included 586 patients with diabetes with a previous MI and LDL cholesterol concentration of 3–4.5 mmol/l. Compared with placebo, a daily dose of 40 mg pravastatin over five years produced relative risks of 0.75 (p = 0.05) for all CAD events and 0.68 (p = 0.04) for revascularization procedures.[161] The results in terms of relative risk reductions in the diabetic and non-diabetic subgroups in both studies were similar. Because patients with diabetes had a higher risk of events they gained more in terms of absolute benefit.

Heart Protection Study (HPS)

The results of these studies in secondary prevention of CAD have recently been supported by the results of the much larger HPS.[162] In this UK Medical Research Council/British Heart Foundation study, 20,536 patients aged 40–80 years with total cholesterol concentration >3.5 mmol/l were randomized to 40 mg simvastatin daily or placebo. Of those randomized, 14,537 had a history of CVD but no diabetes and 5963 had diabetes, both entry criteria identifying patients with an increased risk of atherosclerotic events. In the subgroup with diabetes, 2912 patients had no previous history of arterial disease. Among the patients with diabetes, over a mean follow-up period of 4.8 years, there was a 27% reduction in major coronary events (12.6 versus 9.4%; p <0.0001), a 20% reduction in coronary mortality (8% versus 6.5%; p = 0.02) and a 24% reduction in stroke (5.5 versus 3.5%; p = 0.0002).[163]

The same benefit was seen in the primary and secondary prevention groups, in all age groups and in those with a baseline LDL cholesterol <3.0 mmol/l. After making allowances for non-compliance, it was calculated that the use of simvastatin would reduce the risk of first major vascular events by about one-third. Importantly, the risks of first and subsequent events were reduced. The investigators estimated that treatment with simvastatin for five years would prevent 30 major cardiovascular events in patients with diabetes who had no prior evidence of occlusive vascular disease. Antioxidants were ineffective in the HPS, with little evidence of benefit in other major trials.[164]

Other studies that included subgroups of patients with diabetes have included the following.

The Antihypertensive and Lipid-Lowering Treatment to Prevent Heart Attack Trial (ALLHAT)

The lipid-lowering arm of ALLHAT[165] comprised a subset of patients aged ≥55 years participating in this trial of hypertensive agents with moderately elevated cholesterol levels randomized to pravastatin 40 mg daily (n = 5170) or to usual care (n = 5185), of whom 35% had type 2 diabetes. Mean follow up was 4.8 years. During the trial, 32% of usual care participants with CAD and 29% without started taking lipid-lowering drugs. All-cause mortality was similar for the two groups (relative risk 0.99; 95% confidence interval 0.89–1.11; p = 0.88), with six-year mortality rates of 14.9% for pravastatin versus 15.3% with usual care. Coronary event rates were not significantly different between the groups (relative risk 0.91; 95% confidence interval 0.79–1.04; p = 0.16). The modest differential in total cholesterol (9.6%) and LDL cholesterol (16.7%) between pravastatin and usual care was suggested to be the reason for the lack of benefit observed in this study.

The Anglo-Scandinavian Cardiac Outcomes Trial – Lipid Lowering Arm (ASCOT-LLA)

ASCOT-LLA[166] comprised a subgroup of 10,305 of patients in the main trial comparing antihypertensive therapies with non-fasting total cholesterol concentrations 6.5 mmol/l. Patients were randomly assigned additional atorvastatin 10 mg or placebo. Follow up for an average of five years was planned, the primary end point being non-fatal MI and fatal CAD. Treatment was stopped after a median follow up of 3.3 years. Atorvastatin lowered total serum cholesterol by about 1.3 mmol/l compared with placebo at 12 months, and by 1.1 mmol/l after three years of follow up. By the time the study was terminated, 100 primary events had occurred in the atorvastatin group compared with 154 events in the placebo group (hazard ratio 0.64; 95% confidence interval 0.50–0.83; p = 0.0005). This benefit emerged in the first year of follow up. Although the unadjusted hazard ratio for the subgroup with diabetes (n = 2532) was 0.84, it was not statistically significant (95% confidence interval 0.55–1.29). The low number of events, allied to the foreshortened study period, probably served to reduce the power of the study with respect to the diabetic subgroup.

The Collaborative Atorvastatin Diabetes Study (CARDS)

CARDS[167] was the first primary prevention study of statin therapy conducted exclusively in patients with type 2 diabetes. Some 2838 patients aged 40–75 years with type 2 diabetes and no history of CVD were randomized to placebo (n = 1410) or atorvastatin 10 mg daily (n = 1428). Patients had an LDL cholesterol concentration ≤4.14 mmol/l, fasting triglyceride ≤6.78 mmol/l, and one or more of the following: retinopathy, albuminuria, being a current smoker or hypertension. The pre-specified early stopping rule for efficacy was met two years earlier than planned; median follow up was 3.9 years.

During this period, 127 patients allocated placebo (2.46 per 100 person-years at risk) and 83 allocated atorvastatin (1.54 per 100 person-years at risk) had at least one major cardiovascular event (rate reduction 37%; 95% confidence interval −52 to −17; p = 0.001). Treatment would be expected to prevent at least 37 and 46 major vascular events per 1000 such people treated for four and five years, respectively. Assessed separately, acute coronary arterial disease events were reduced by 36% (−55 to −9), coronary revascularization procedures by 31% (−59 to 16), and rate of stroke by 48% (−69 to −11). Atorvastatin reduced the death rate by 27% (−48 to 1; p = 0.059). No excess of adverse events was noted in the atorvastatin group.

So, should all patients with type 2 diabetes now be treated with a statin as a primary prevention measure? As discussed earlier, this view is not universally accepted, with some authorities continuing to argue the case for calculating the overall cardiovascular risk of the individual patient.[27]

Fibrates

The typical patient with type 2 diabetes will have total and LDL cholesterol concentrations that reflect the background non-diabetic population. However, this will frequently be associated with small, dense LDL cholesterol and a reduced HDL cholesterol concentration. The prevalence of hypertriglyceridaemia in type 2 diabetes is two to three times higher than in non-diabetics.[168] The fibrates represent a logical choice for these patients. However, while several placebo-controlled trials have reported reductions in coronary events in non-diabetic and diabetic patients using fibrates, the current evidence is less rigorous than the evidence supporting the use of statins.

Helsinki Heart Study

This placebo-controlled study of 4081 men included a small number (n =135) with diabetes. A non-significant reduction in CAD was observed in patients with diabetes treated with gemfibrozil (3.4% versus 10.5%).[169] The coronary event and death rates were higher in the patients with diabetes than in the non-diabetic participants, the former group having more hypertension and a higher prevalence of the aforementioned dyslipidaemia. When the entire placebo group of the trial (n = 2045) was analysed, the combination of hypertriglyceridaemia

(>2.3 mmol/l) in concert with a ratio of LDL to HDL >5 was the best predictor of cardiac events.[170]

Veterans Administration High Density lipoprotein Intervention Trial (VA-HIT)[171]

This secondary prevention trial included 2531 men with CAD and low levels of HDL cholesterol. Patients with diabetes comprised 25% of the total; mean baseline HDL cholesterol concentration was 0.8 mmol/l. A reduction in combined non-fatal and fatal coronary events (22%; p = 0.006) and stroke (27%; p = 0.05) was observed with gemfibrozil. Of interest, the benefits of gemfibrozil appeared to be more dependent on the presence of insulin resistance than baseline lipid levels.[172]

> *Reducing LDL cholesterol levels is currently regarded as the primary therapeutic aim of lipid–lowering therapy*

Diabetes Atherosclerosis Intervention Study (DAIS)

DAIS examined the effects of fenofibrate or placebo on the progression of CAD in 418 patients with type 2 diabetes with dyslipidaemia.[173] Fenofibrate was associated with a 6% increase in HDL cholesterol, a 28% decrease in triglycerides and a 5% decrease in LDL cholesterol. Although a significant 40% reduction in the progression of focal coronary lesions with fenofibrate 200 mg daily was observed, the trial was not sufficiently powered to reliably demonstrate a significant reduction (23%) in clinical events. It is unclear whether a 55% increase in plasma homocysteine (see section on *Cardiovascular risk factors in the patient with diabetes*) might have detracted from the benefits of the drug.

Therapeutic targets

The results of interventional clinical trials using statins strongly favour lowering the concentration of LDL cholesterol as the principal aim of therapy. The HPS extended this approach to patients with pretreatment cholesterol levels previously regarded as targets for intervention, rather than thresholds for treatment. Therefore, the maxim, with some caveats, has become to use statins in patients at high risk whose pretreatment LDL cholesterol is >3.5 mmol/l. In such circumstances, the 2004 British guidelines suggest lowering total cholesterol by 25%, or <4.0 mmol/l, or LDL cholesterol by 30%, or <2.0 mmol/l, whichever is greater.[25,174] This applies to patients at least until age 80 years.

A recent update of the NCEP guidelines suggests that even more intensive therapy might be indicated for patients at highest risk, such as those with diabetes who have occlusive CVD; a target of <1.8 mmol/l has been proposed.[175] Apolipoprotein B levels (see section on *Cardiovascular risk factors in the patient with diabetes*) are regarded as

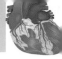

being near optimal at this concentration of LDL cholesterol. The 2005 ADA guidelines[176] include updated recommendations:

- In patients with diabetes aged >40 years with a total cholesterol ≥3.5 mmol/l, without overt cardiovascular disease, statin therapy is recommended to achieve an LDL cholesterol reduction of 30–40%, irrespective of baseline levels. The primary goal is an LDL cholesterol <2.6 mmol/l
- For patients aged <40 years without overt CVD but at increased risk (due to other cardiovascular risk factors or long duration of diabetes), who do not achieve lipid goals with lifestyle modifications alone, the addition of pharmacological therapy is appropriate and the primary goal is an LDL cholesterol <2.6 mmol/l
- A lower LDL cholesterol goal of <1.8 mmol/l, using a high dose of a statin, is an option in high-risk patients with diabetes and overt CVD.

All patients with diabetes with cardiovascular disease should receive lipid-lowering therapy (usually with a statin) if there is no contra-indication

Part of the controversy about lipid targets revolves around the issue of whether the level of LDL cholesterol is the only mechanism of benefit.[177] Recent data support the view that statins can improve clinical outcomes via reduced inflammation – an effect that is independent of reductions in cholesterol levels.[178] Studies of new drugs with different mechanisms of action, such as the intestinal cholesterol uptake inhibitor ezetimibe,[179] may help to resolve this issue as well as offering an alternative to high-dose statins. Beneficial effects of statins on aspects of renal function may be relevant to reducing the risk of CVD in patients with proteinuria.[180]

Some of the evidence for this new low target level comes from studies in patients with acute coronary syndromes such as the Pravastatin or Atorvastatin Evaluation and Infection Therapy–Thrombolysis in Myocardial Infarction study (PROVE-IT).[181] This study, like the Myocardial Ischemia Reduction with Aggressive Cholesterol Lowering (MIRACL) trial, showed rapid onset of benefits from high-dose atorvastatin.[182] The high toll among patients with diabetes and stable CVD provides a rationale for intensive statin therapy. Certainly, current strategies leave many patients at risk of recurrent vascular events. The issue of titrating to target levels of lipids is likely to be further fuelled by the results of ongoing studies, in which more aggressive lipid goals are being studied.

In some circumstances, statin–fibrate combination therapy may be considered when targets are not reached with either drug alone. Although generally well tolerated, this combination is currently outside licence restrictions; expert advice should be sought. Concerns about the safety of statin–fibrate therapy have recently been fuelled by an increased risk of adverse events reported with gemfibrozil, relative to

Combined statin–fibrate therapy carries increased risks; expert advice should be sought

fenofibrate. This was predominantly manifested as an increased rate of rhabdomyolysis in patients taking the combination of gemfibrozil and a statin, particularly cerivastatin.[183] The latter drug was withdrawn in the US and Europe in 2001.

Cautions and contraindications

Statins and fibrates are generally well tolerated. Doses of fibrates should be reduced in patients with minor degrees of renal impairment; they should not be avoided in moderate and severe renal failure. The issue of whether fibrates or statins should be used in unexplained hepatic impairment or active liver disease is contentious. Current licences caution against using these drugs in such circumstances; expert advice should be sought. When considering prescribing statins, it is important to consider the potential for drug interactions. This is particularly pertinent in patients with diabetes who are likely to be treated with multiple classes of drugs.

> *Fibrates should not be used in renal failure*

- Decreased statin metabolism – azole antifungals (itraconazole and ketoconazole), macrolides such as erythromycin and clarithromycin, calcium-channel blockers (particularly verapamil and diltiazem), cyclosporin and grapefruit juice potentially increase plasma levels of other statins by inhibiting hepatic metabolism, and may enhance the risk of myositis when dyslipidaemia is treated with atorvastatin, lovastatin or simvastatin. Potential alternative agents are pravastatin (extrahepatic metabolism), fluvastatin (metabolized by the CYP2C9 isoenzyme of the cytochrome P450 enzyme system) or rosuvastatin.

> *All statins except pravastatin may enhance the effects of warfarin – close monitoring is necessary*

- Potentiation of other drugs – careful monitoring of anticoagulation is needed when starting any hepatically metabolized statin in patients treated with warfarin, because the effect of the anticoagulant may be increased.

Recent developments and emerging therapies for dyslipidaemia

Several new approaches to lipid modification have been developed in recent years. These include:

- Ezetimibe – this intestinal cholesterol absorption inhibitor introduced in 2003 offers a new approach to reducing LDL cholesterol levels.[184] Ezetimibe may be used either as monotherapy or in conjunction with statins. A combination preparation of ezetimibe with simvastatin in ratios from 10:10 to 10:80 is available in some counties
- Agents that raise HDL cholesterol – over the next few years, it seems likely that, in addition to a continuing debate about optimal levels of LDL cholesterol, attention will be directed to raising HDL

cholesterol. Of the currently available drugs, nicotinic acid (niacin) preparations are regarded as being most effective. However, the use of these preparations is often limited by facial flushing.[179] A new approach to raising HDL levels is inhibition of cholesteryl ester transfer protein (see section on *Cardiovascular risk factors in the patient with diabetes*).[185] With some theoretical provisos about this approach,[186] drugs such as torcetrapib offer a means of favourably influencing a major facet of diabetic dyslipidaemia[187]

- Omega-3 fatty acids – recent clinical trial data, including studies using the concentrated omega-3 fatty acid preparation Omacor, indicate that omega-3 fatty acids can prevent sudden death following MI.[188] Omega-3 fatty acids are as effective as, or have a benefit superior to, statins in secondary prevention. Omacor is also useful in the treatment of hypertriglyceridaemia, both as monotherapy and in combination with statins.

High blood pressure

Recent clinical trials have informed target blood pressures and have helped to clarify the issue of which drugs are most advantageous in the diabetic patient. Shared conclusions of these studies include:

- Two or more drugs from different classes are needed to achieve blood pressure targets in many patients
- The principal consideration is the level of blood pressure attained, rather than the selection of drugs with particular modes of action.

Note that despite the sound evidence base, under-treatment of hypertension is common in both non-diabetic and diabetic populations. As far as targets are concerned, the general trend in recent years has been a steady reduction. Bear in mind that targets that seem near-impossible to attain in many patients should be distinguished from acceptable levels of control attained in most patients in practice. Unfortunately, discrepancies in recommendations between expert groups are not infrequently encountered. Although these are not usually dramatic, they can cause a sense of unease among clinicians responsible for managing these challenging patients.

Evidence for treating hypertension in diabetes

Key clinical trials that have informed the treatment of hypertension in patients with diabetes include the following.

Systolic Hypertension in the Elderly Program (SHEP)

In a subgroup of patients with diabetes (583 patients out of a total of 4736), treatment for five years with chlorthalidone, plus atenolol or reserpine if needed, produced an average fall in seated blood pressure

83

of around 10/2 mmHg relative to placebo.[189] This resulted in significant reductions in major cardiovascular events, i.e. non-fatal MI, fatal CAD and major CAD events, with trends towards reductions in both stroke and all-cause mortality. Absolute risk reduction with active treatment, compared with placebo, was twice as great for diabetic versus non-diabetic patients (101/1000 versus 51/1000 randomized participants at the five-year follow up), reflecting the higher risk of diabetic patients.

Systolic Hypertension-Europe (SYST-EUR)

Similar results were seen in this study, in which patients were randomized to placebo or nitrendipine, with the addition of enalapril or hydrochlorthiazide if blood pressure targets were not reached.[190] An average fall in blood pressure of 10.1/4.5 mmHg for two years resulted in a significant fall in total strokes (relative risk 0.58; 95% confidence interval 0.4–0.83; p = 0.003), non-fatal stroke (relative risk 0.56; 95% confidence interval 0.37–0.86; p = 0.007), all fatal and non-fatal cardiac end points (relative risk 0.74; 95% confidence interval 0.47–0.97; p = 0.03) and all fatal and non-fatal cardiovascular end points (relative risk 0.69; 95% confidence interval 0.55–0.86; p <0.001). Some 492 patients out of a total of 4695 had diabetes, the end point reductions being greater in the diabetic subgroup than in the study population as a whole (stroke: relative risk 0.31; 95% confidence interval 0.11–0.88; p = 0.02; all cardiovascular events: relative risk 0.38; 95% confidence interval 0.2–0.81; p = 0.002; all cardiac events: relative risk 0.43; 95% confidence interval 0.18–1.06; p = 0.06).

These studies established that blood pressure lowering in diabetes improves long-term outcomes. However, they did not establish the optimal drug treatment or the most appropriate blood pressure targets.

Hypertension in Diabetes Study (HDS)

In 1987, a randomized study of blood pressure control (published as UKPDS 38 and 39)[191,156] was embedded within the main glycaemic control study of the UKPDS in a factorial design. The HDS blood pressure substudy provided important confirmation of the adverse effect of hypertension in patients with type 2 diabetes. A mean blood pressure reduction of 10/5 mmHg between the tight and less tight blood pressure groups resulted in reductions in:

- Diabetes-related end points (relative risk 0.76; 95% confidence interval 0.62–0.92; p = 0.0046)
- Diabetes-related deaths (relative risk 0.68; 95% confidence interval 0.49–0.94; p = 0.019)

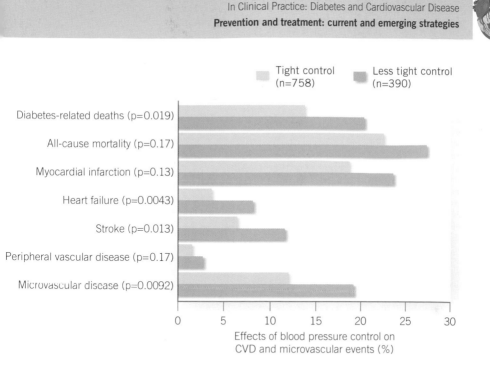

Figure 28. Data from
United Kingdom
Prospective Diabetes
Study 38. Tight blood
pressure control and risk
of macrovascular and
microvascular
complications in type 2
diabetes: UKPDS 38
(CVD = cardiovascular
disease). *BMJ*
1998;317:703–713.

- Microvascular end points (relative risk 0.63; 95% confidence interval 0.44–0.89; p = 0.0092).

Among single end points, there were clinically relevant reductions in progression of retinopathy (relative risk 0.66; 99% confidence interval 0.50–0.89; p = 0.0038), fatal and non-fatal stroke (relative risk for latter 0.56; 99% confidence interval 0.28–1.12; p = 0.013) and cardiac failure (relative risk 0.44; 99% confidence interval 0.20–0.94; p = 0.0043), although a 21% reduction in MI was not statistically significant (Figure 28). Tight blood pressure control produced benefits in both microvascular and CVD end points that exceeded those observed through improved glycaemic control.

Although the study had captopril- and atenolol-treatment arms, it was not sufficiently powered to differentiate between these treatments. However, some differences between these drugs were evident. Captopril was better tolerated than atenolol, with 78% versus 65% of patients still taking their allocated drug at their last clinic visit (p <0.0001). Patients randomized to atenolol gained more body weight and needed higher doses of antidiabetic medication compared with those receiving captopril. From the analysis of the UKPDS cohort, it has been estimated that each 10 mmHg drop in mean systolic blood pressure is associated with reductions of:

- 12% for any diabetes-related complication
- 15% in deaths related to diabetes
- 11% in MI
- 13% in microvascular complications.

Around one-third of patients needed three or more antihypertensive drugs to achieve moderate blood pressure control, with only 56% reaching target in the so-called 'tight' blood pressure control arm.

Hypertension Optimal Treatment (HOT)

In this study, 18,790 patients with hypertension and a diastolic blood pressure of 100–115 mmHg were randomized to one of three groups, aiming for a target diastolic blood pressure of ≤90 mmHg, ≤85 mmHg or ≤80 mmHg (achieved blood pressures: 85.2, 83.2 and 81.1 mmHg, respectively).[192] Felodipine was used as first-line therapy and was titrated according to a predetermined algorithm. Half the patients were also randomly assigned to receive aspirin (75 mg/day).

In the study population as a whole, there were no significant differences in outcomes between the blood pressure target groups. However, in the subgroup of 1501 patients with diabetes, the risk of major cardiovascular events and mortality were significantly lower in the ≤80 mmHg target group, compared with the ≤90 mmHg target group (11.9 versus 24.4 events/1000 patient years; p = 0.005 and 3.7 versus 11.1 events/1000 patient years; p = 0.016, respectively). For major cardiovascular events, the lowest risk was at a mean achieved pressure of 138.5/82.6 mmHg. For stroke, the corresponding value was 142/80 mmHg.

ALLHAT

In ALLHAT[193] 33,357 patients older than 55 years with hypertension and one other risk factor for CAD risk were randomized to blood pressure regimens based on chlorthalidone (n = 15,255), amlodipine (n = 9048) or lisinopril (n = 9054). During a mean follow up of 4.9 years, there were no differences between groups in the primary end point of fatal CAD or non-fatal MI. In an analysis of predefined secondary end points, heart failure was more common in the amlodipine group compared with the chlorthalidone group (10.2% versus 7.7%; relative risk 1.38; 95% confidence interval 1.25–1.52). Combined CVD events (i.e. combined CAD, stroke, treated angina without hospitalization, heart failure and peripheral arterial disease), heart failure and stroke were more common in the lisinopril group than the chlorthalidone group. As with the total study population, there were

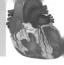

no differences in the primary end point between groups in the 15,297 patients who had diabetes.

Therefore, no major advantage was observed between more traditional, i.e. diuretic-based therapy, and either a calcium antagonist or ACE inhibitor. Despite its impressive size, this study has attracted criticism for perceived failings, for example low rates of continuation on allocated therapy and differences in attained blood pressure between groups, which have detracted from the reliability of the conclusions relating to particular end points. Moreover, results obtained using chlorthalidone, a relatively potent long-acting thiazide-like diuretic, might not be able to be extrapolated to thiazides.

There have been three recent large studies that have suggested that ACE inhibitors and ARBs may have effects that extend beyond blood pressure lowering in selected patients with and without diabetes. However, some of the differences between the outcomes in these reports and the results of ALLHAT may relate to the particular patient groups included or other methodological issues. Whether intrinsic properties of the drugs explained the entirety of the benefits, as opposed to reductions in blood pressure, has been debated.

> *The extent of blood pressure lowering and target achieved appear more important than the class of drug used*

Heart Outcomes Prevention Evaluation (HOPE)
In this study, 9297 high-risk patients aged 55 years or older with evidence of vascular disease or diabetes and one other cardiovascular risk factor (cholesterol >5.2 mmol/l, HDL cholesterol <0.9mmol/l, hypertension, microalbuminuria or current smoker), were randomized to either 10 mg ramipril daily or placebo, in addition to other medication for a median of 4.5 years.[194] Patients in each group took other cardiovascular medication, including treatment for hypertension.

Treatment with ramipril reduced the rates of cardiovascular death (6.1% versus 8.1%; relative risk 0.74; p <0.001), MI (9.9% versus 12.3%; relative risk 0.8; p <0.001) and stroke (3.4% versus 4.9%; relative risk 0.68; p <0.001). The study included 3577 patients with diabetes, and the results for that group were reported separately.[195] The risk reductions were similar, with a 22% reduction in MI, a 33% reduction in stroke and a 37% reduction in total mortality. After adjusting for the mean blood pressure difference of 2.4/1.0 mmHg between the ramipril and the placebo groups, there was no change in the main findings of the study.

Following the publication of these studies, the UK licence for ramipril was extended for diabetic patients older than 55 years with additional risk factors for CVD. However, there has been much discussion about the difference in blood pressure between the groups and how important this might be in explaining the results. A subgroup of patients on ramipril who underwent 24-hour blood pressure monitoring showed improvements in blood pressure that were not evident from the clinic blood pressure measurements. Accordingly, it has been suggested that this may explain the differences between the ramipril and placebo groups rather than any putative non-blood pressure lowering effects of ramipril.

Losartan Intervention For Endpoint in hypertension (LIFE)

This study included 1195 patients with diabetes, hypertension and left ventricular hypertrophy on electrocardiographic criteria, who were randomized to losartan-based or atenolol-based blood pressure lowering treatment.[196] After a mean follow up of nearly five years, death from CVD was reduced in the losartan group (6% versus 10%; relative risk 0.63; p = 0.028) as was all-cause mortality (11% versus 17%; relative risk 0.61; p = 0.002). The difference in blood pressure between groups was minor − 2/0 mmHg in favour of losartan at the end of the study. The benefits of losartan in this study were largely driven by a 25% reduction in stroke in the main study.

EUROpean trial on reduction of cardiac events with Perindopril in stable coronary Artery disease (EUROPA)

This trial included 12,218 patients with stable CAD who were randomized to either perindopril 8 mg daily or placebo for just over four years.[197] The primary end point (cardiovascular mortality, non-fatal MI or resuscitated arrest) occurred in 10% of patients on placebo and 8% on perindopril (relative risk 0.8; p = 0.0003). The study included 1502 patients with diabetes, of whom 721 were randomized to perindopril.

The relative risk reductions were similar in this group to the entire study population but with the smaller sample size reducing the power, statistical significance was not reached. There was a small blood pressure difference between the perindopril and placebo treatment groups.

Prevention of Events with Angiotensin Converting Enzyme inhibitor trial (PEACE)

This study provided evidence that countered the view that all patients with CAD should receive an ACE inhibitor. In patients with preserved left ventricular function on current standard therapy, no benefit was seen from adding trandolapril.[198] However, it has been suggested that the study may have been underpowered. It could be argued that higher risk patients with diabetes might be most likely to derive benefit from such an approach.[199]

The results of the LIFE study notwithstanding, the most compelling reason to consider using ARBs in patients with type 2 diabetes rests on recent short-term studies of inpatients with

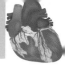

End point	IDNT (irbesartan vs amlodipine)	IDNT (amlodipine vs placebo)	RENAAL (losartan vs placebo)	IRMA-2 (irbesartan vs placebo)
2 x Creatinine level	37% (p <0.001)	–6% (p = 0.60)	25% (p = 0.006)	33% (p = 0.03)
2 x Creatinine level, ESRD or death	23% (p = 0.006)	–4% (p = 0.69)	16% (p = 0.02)	20% (p = 0.02)
ESRD	23% (p = 0.07)	0% (p = 0.99)	28% (p = 0.002)	23% (p = 0.07)
Death	–4% (p = 0.8)	12% (p = 0.4)	–2% (p = 0.88)	8% (p = 0.57)
Cardiovascular morbidity and mortality	–3% (p = 0.79)	12% (p = 0.29)	10% (p = 0.26)	9% (p = 0.4)

CHD = coronary heart disease; ESRD = end-stage renal disease; IDNT = Irbesartan Diabetic Nephropathy Trial; IRMA-2 = Irbesartan Microalbuminuria 2 Trial; RENAAL = Reduction in End Points in NIDDM with the Angiotensin II Antagonist Losartan study

Table 20. Relative risk reductions in angiotensin receptor blocker studies. **Reproduced with permission from Sowers JR. Treatment of hypertension in patients with diabetes.** *Arch Intern Med* 2004;164:1850–1857. Copyright © 2001 American Medical Association. All rights reserved.

nephropathy.[98] Although these studies showed that progression of diabetic nephropathy can be favourably altered through the use of ARBs, none had adequate statistical power to demonstrate a reduction in cardiovascular events (Table 20). Few studies have compared ARBs with ACE inhibitors. In a comparative study in patients with type 2 diabetes and early nephropathy, telmisartan at 80 mg daily appeared to be as effective as enalapril 20 mg daily on glomerular filtration rate over five years.[200] ACE inhibition can prevent the development of microalbuminuria in patients with type 2 diabetes and normal urinary albumin excretion[201,202]

There have been consistent reports from recent randomized clinical trials of anti-diabetic effects of drugs that interrupt the renin–angiotensin system.[203] However, new-onset diabetes was not a pre-specified end point in any of these trials. A meta-analysis of seven studies showed that ACE inhibitors and ARBs decreased new diabetes by 20%, compared with diuretics and ß-blockers (p <0.001). Calcium channel blockers decreased new diabetes by 16% (p <0.001). When compared with placebo, ramipril and candesartan, both decreased the incidence of new diabetes (see below: ASCOT).

These data raise the possibility that these agents prevent the changes leading to insulin resistance; attenuation of the adverse effects of angiotensin II on the endothelium has been postulated. These intriguing observations might provide a basis for novel strategies to

89

prevent type 2 diabetes in high-risk patients using drugs with proven efficacy in CVD. Postulated mechanisms include:

- Improved whole body insulin sensitivity
- Lowered circulating fatty acid concentrations
- Increased adiponectin concentrations – this effect has been reported for some types of ARBs.

Other postulated mechanisms include attenuation of sympathetic overactivity, effects on the islet microvasculature with improved islet β-cell function, and alterations in skeletal muscle fibre composition. Shared cellular effects of angiotensin II and insulin that are mediated through insulin receptor substrate-1 are of interest in this regard. There are increasing data suggesting that angiotensin II, acting through its type 1 receptor, inhibits insulin action in vascular and skeletal muscle tissue. In part, this appears to be due to interference of insulin signalling through the phosphatidylinositol 3-kinase pathway. The end result is decreased endothelial cell production of nitric oxide and increased myosin light chain activation with vasoconstriction, and reduced skeletal muscle glucose transport.[204]

Thiazide diuretics and especially β-blockers may impair whole body insulin sensitivity and predispose to development of diabetes.[205] Non-randomized studies have suggested an additive effect of the combination on risk of developing type 2 diabetes. As might be expected, new-onset diabetes appears to be associated with increased CVD risk.[206] Adverse effects on lipids and hypokalaemia are other unwelcome effects of the older agents. In 2005 preliminary results of the aforementioned ASCOT study were announced (Sever P. and Dahlof B., American College of Cardiology, Orlando, March 2005). The study, which enrolled 19,257 hypertensive patients, aged 40 to 79 years, with no previous MI or clinical CAD, was terminated early because the reduction in stroke (23%, p<0.001), total coronary events (14%, p=0.005), cardiovascular death (24%, p<0.001) and all-cause mortality (14%, p<0.001) was greater in the amlodipine/perindopril arm compared with the β-blocker/diuretic arm. New-onset diabetes was reduced by 32% (p<0.001).

Two large, prospective, placebo-controlled randomized clinical trials are under way whose primary outcome is the prevention of type 2 diabetes: DREAM, NAVIGATOR and the ONgoing Telmisartan Alone and in combination with Ramipril Global Endpoint Trial (ONTARGET) will investigate as a secondary end point whether it is possible to prevent the development of type 2 diabetes by blocking the renin–angiotensin system with either an ACE inhibitor or an ARB, or a combination.[203]

As for other drugs, moxonidine, which selectively targets imidazo-line type-1 receptors in the sympathetic vasomotor centres of the rostral-ventrolateral medulla, has been reported to exert favourable metabolic effects in preclinical and clinical studies.[207] Comparative studies with ACE inhibitors are in progress.

Strategies for managing hypertension in diabetes
Non-pharmacological measures

These are regarded as the cornerstone of therapy. These measures, the benefits of which are often underestimated and rarely attained, include:

- Reduction in body weight for patients who are overweight or obese
- Reduced dietary salt intake – this is an important, and perhaps underappreciated, aspect of management in patients eating typical Western high-salt diets; salt substitutes may be helpful
- Increased potassium intake, through eating fresh fruit and vegetables
- Aerobic physical exercise – for example, brisk walking for a total of 30 minutes or more daily, or suitable alternative activity.

Reductions in blood pressure with therapeutic lifestyle measures of around 5 mmHg or greater may be possible with 10 kg weight reduction and increased levels of regular physical exertion. Compromises are often necessary, i.e. partial weight reduction rather than attaining ideal body weight, or even preventing further weight gain. This advice should be periodically reinforced, unless inappropriate for an individual patient.

If drug therapy proves necessary, which will be the case for most patients, non-pharmacological measures can be useful for limiting the need for medication. Not all such measures will be appropriate for every patient.

Drug therapy

In patients without severe uncontrolled hypertension, which demands prompt treatment, several readings of blood over a few weeks should be used to inform the decision to start treatment. Blood pressure should be measured annually in all adult patients with diabetes. If end-organ damage is present, for example left ventricular hypertrophy or proteinuria, or blood pressure exceeds 160/100 mmHg, treatment should start with the most appropriate first-line drug. For other patients, if blood pressure exceeds 140/80 mmHg it should be rechecked on two or three occasions to establish the baseline before starting treatment.

Several studies have shown that both tight glycaemic control and blood pressure control can improve urinary albumin excretion in patients with type 2 diabetes. Recent results with thiazolidinediones have led to speculation that these drugs may be beneficial for achieving glucose control and reducing the development or worsening of microalbuminuria or hypertension.[208]

The 2004 ADA guidelines,[209] 2004 BHS[25,174] and the Joint National Committee 7th Report[103] recommend a systolic target based largely on epidemiological data of <130/80 mmHg for patients with diabetes. The ADA recommends using an ACE inhibitor or ARB as first-line therapy. For patients with nephropathy who are unable to take one of these agents, non-dihydropyridine calcium channel blockers, such as verapamil or diltiazem, are preferred to dihydropyridines; the latter class is not effective for slowing the progression of nephropathy. In practice, a low-dose diuretic would be first choice for many physicians. Drugs should be substituted or added in logical combinations (for example an ACE inhibitor and thiazide diuretic, or long-acting calcium antagonist).

The BHS has modified and approved an algorithm for treating hypertension based on an 'AB/CD' rule; the 'AB' category lowers blood pressure via suppression of the renin–angiotensin system.

- *Step1*: For younger (<55 years) and non-black patients, start with either an ACE inhibitor or ARB (A) or β-blocker (B). For older or black patients, start with a (long-acting) calcium channel blocker (C) or thiazide diuretic (D).
- *Step 2*: Add A (or B) + C or D.

Table 21. Indications for particular antihypertensive drugs in diabetic patients.

Indication	Drugs of choice
Nephropathy	ACE inhibitors (+ loop diuretics) Angiotensin receptor blockers Non-dihydropyridine calcium antagonists
Ischaemic heart disease	Beta-blockers Long-acting calcium antagonists; avoid combination of rate-limiting drugs such as verapamil and diltiazem with beta-blockers – risk of bradycardia or heart block
Cardiac failure	Diuretics; loop diuretics, e.g. furosemide – may require high doses if renal impairment is present ACE inhibitors Angiotensin receptor blockers Beta-blockers; certain drugs, e.g. carvedilol in selected patients with stable heart failure

ACE = angiotensin converting enzyme

- *Step 3*: Use A + B + C. In non-diabetic patients the combination of thiazide + β-blocker is not recommended because of the possible increased risk of diabetes (see above).
- *Step 4*: Add an α-blocker or spironolactone or another diuretic, such as a loop diuretic. In our experience, moxonidine can also be useful as third- or fourth-line agent in selected patients.

Use low doses of each agent to minimize unwanted effects. Other practical points include:

- Co-morbidities – some patients may have compelling indications (Table 21) for certain drugs because of co-morbidities commonly associated with diabetes
- Thiazide or thiazide-like diuretics – these are often useful because hypertension in patients with diabetes may be associated with an expanded plasma volume
- Loop diuretics – often necessary for patients with significant renal impairment in whom hypertension is often difficult to control.

As already mentioned, multiple-drug regimens are often needed in the pursuit of ever more challenging targets. Initiating drug therapy with two agents may be appropriate for patients with blood pressure >20/10 mmHg above goal. Patients with diabetes often need many drugs – oral antidiabetic agents, lipid-lowering agents, aspirin and so on – which creates problems for long-term compliance, as well as increasing the chances of adverse interactions.

Because hypertension is largely asymptomatic, once-daily dosing and using well-tolerated drugs are likely to improve adherence to therapy. The ARBs appear to be particularly well-tolerated agents; they do not share the propensity to cause the unproductive cough that is induced in a substantial minority of patients treated with ACE inhibitors. However, these agents are more expensive than diuretics, which is an important consideration in what is usually life-long therapy.

Clinical trials suggest that patients of African descent with hypertension, who tend to have low plasma renin levels, respond better to β-blockers and calcium antagonists than to ACE inhibitors. This is taken into account in the 'AB/CD' rule discussed above. The 'CD' agents tend to raise renin concentrations, thereby providing a substrate for the 'AB' category of drugs. South Asian patients, who often have appreciable insulin resistance, respond well to metabolically neutral ACE inhibitors. However, given the likelihood of multiple drugs being needed to achieve targets, theoretical concerns about metabolically disadvantageous effects should not be used to deny medication with proven benefit to patients with diabetes.

Do certain antihypertensive agents offer advantages?

This issue has been debated in relation to the perceived shortfall in reducing the risk of MI using older classes of antihypertensive agents. The data from recent comparative studies involving large numbers of patients generally do not provide support for major drug-specific benefits. The controversy about the HOPE study has already been discussed.

Although a minor advantage has been observed with calcium channel blockers for reducing strokes, this only just reaches statistical significance in meta-analyses. Conversely, calcium channel blockers may be less effective than other agents at preventing MI; differences in attained blood pressure with different drugs in clinical trials complicate these issues. Concerns about inferiority of certain calcium blockers compared with other agents – derived in the case of diabetes from some underpowered studies lacking placebo control groups – have largely evaporated in recent years. Short-acting calcium antagonists, however, are not recommended. Some studies have suggested that ARBs, ACE inhibitors and some calcium antagonists reduce left ventricular hypertrophy more effectively than β-blockers at similar levels of blood pressure control.

Cautions and contraindications

Diabetic patients are at risk of developing long-term tissue complications, which may render certain choices of antihypertensive drugs unsuitable (Table 22). Treatment of hypertension in patients with diabetes may also be complicated by other considerations.

- Risk of hypoglycaemia – problems with impaired recognition of warning symptoms and recovery of blood glucose levels from hypoglycaemia are uncommon with more modern cardioselective β-blockers, such as atenolol. Insulin treatment should not be regarded as a contraindication to the use of such drugs, which confer benefit to diabetic patients, especially following MI. In the hypertension substudy of the UKPDS, there was no difference in the risk of severe hypoglycaemia between the atenolol- and captopril-based treatment groups. Hypoglycaemia associated with ACE inhibitors, which are credited with minor beneficial effects on insulin action, appears to be uncommon in the UK despite reports of an association.
- Risks associated with renal artery stenosis – a minority of patients with type 2 diabetes with peripheral arterial disease will also have clinically significant renal artery stenosis. Certain drugs (ACE inhibitors and ARBs) should be used with caution: there is a risk of precipitating an acute deterioration in renal function. If there are functional stenoses of both renal arteries, glomerular filtration is maintained by the vasoconstrictor effect of angiotensin II on efferent

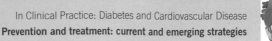

Caution or contraindication	Drugs
Dyslipidaemia	Beta-blockers Thiazides (at higher doses*)
Erectile dysfunction	Beta-blockers Thiazides
Gout	Thiazides
Peripheral vascular disease	Beta-blockers
Renal artery stenosis	ACE inhibitors Angiotensin receptor blockers
*>2.5 mg bendrofluazide daily	

Table 22. Cautions and contraindications to antihypertensive therapy in diabetic patients.

glomerular arterioles. Removal of this effect by these drugs may cause a significant decrease in glomerular filtration.

- Under certain circumstances, for example patients with congestive cardiac failure or generalized atherosclerosis, deterioration in renal function may be encountered even with unilateral renal artery stenosis. It is prudent to check plasma creatinine and electrolytes within a week of starting ACE inhibitor therapy, and following each increase in dosage. The absence of pedal pulses should alert the clinician to the possibility of renal artery stenosis (see section on *Cardiovascular risk factors in the patient with diabetes*). Patients with bilateral renal stenosis are at risk of acute pulmonary oedema. The investigation of renal artery stenosis in selected patients involves imaging; referral to a clinician with expertise is advised.

- Postural hypotension – autonomic neuropathy, which is often asymptomatic but detectable using non-invasive tests of cardiovascular reflex integrity, for example loss of beat-to-beat heart rate variability during deep breathing, may render patients vulnerable to postural hypotension. Supine and erect blood pressure measurements should be taken. Drugs such as tricyclic antidepressants used for their pain-modulating effects in symptomatic peripheral neuropathy may accentuate the effect of antihypertensive agents.

- Erectile dysfunction – this is a common problem among diabetic patients. Drugs with a propensity to induce erectile impotence, for example thiazide diuretics, are best avoided in these circumstances. Bear in mind reports of cardiovascular deaths in patients using sildenafil in conjunction with nitrates, particularly given the high prevalence of subclinical myocardial ischaemia among people with diabetes.

Coronary artery disease

The major clinical manifestations of CAD are sudden death, angina pectoris and acute coronary syndromes including MI. The implications of diabetes for the coronary vasculature are well recognized by cardiologists. Compared with non-diabetics, the characteristics of coronary lesions in patients with diabetes have several important distinctions:

- More extensive and diffuse atherosclerosis
- More common left main stem disease
- More triple vessel disease
- Smaller vessels containing longer lesions
- Impaired vascular remodelling with greater luminal encroachment
- Impaired collateral vessel formation
- Higher coronary calcification scores.

Add to these a higher complication rate after coronary intervention and re-stenosis rates that are in excess of those in non-diabetics, and the stage is set for the high event rates and poor clinical outcomes that are all too familiar.

The coronary plaque in patients with diabetes seems more liable to rupture owing to a thin fibrous cap, more inflammatory cells and fewer smooth muscle cells. In an atherectomy study the percentage of total area occupied by lipid-rich atheroma was larger in specimens from patients with diabetes than in specimens from patients without diabetes.[210] The percentage of total area occupied by macrophages was larger in specimens from patients with diabetes (22%) than in specimens from patients without diabetes (12%; p = 0.003). The incidence of thrombus was also higher in specimens from patients with diabetes than in specimens from patients without diabetes (62% versus 40%; p = 0.04). Higher circulating levels of inflammatory markers such as C-reactive protein are thought to reflect an active contribution to the process of atherogenesis (see section on *Cardiovascular risk factors in the patient with diabetes*).

The close association between acute coronary syndromes and hyperglycaemia are discussed elsewhere. Patients with diabetes are over-represented in coronary angiography suites. Therefore, 20–30% of patients undergoing angiography have diabetes, a prevalence two- to three-fold higher than in the general population.

Acute myocardial infarction

Even in the modern era of rapid thrombolysis, the mortality rate of patients with diabetes following MI is around two-fold higher than in non-diabetic people.[211] Both immediate in-hospital and late mortality rates are increased. As discussed in the section on *Cardiovascular risk factors in the patient with diabetes*, the incidence of heart failure is high

"Immediate and later mortality rates following myocardial infarction are high in patients with type 2 diabetes"

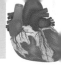

after MI in patients with diabetes. Co-morbidity such as fluid retention and anaemia due to renal impairment contributes to excessive morbidity and mortality rates.

The symptoms of MI may be modified by the presence of diabetes. This implies that the duration of diabetes has been sufficient for chronic complications to develop. So-called clinically 'silent' infarcts are more common in patients with diabetes; neuropathy affecting the autonomic fibres is held to be responsible. Angina pectoris may also be less prominent. The clinical picture is further complicated by the presence of upper gastrointestinal motility problems in some patients that can cause diagnostic difficulties similar symptoms. Acute coronary ischaemia may therefore present atypically with symptoms such as:

- Dyspnoea – this may be accompanied by signs of cardiac failure
- Confusion – particularly in the elderly
- Alterations in glycaemic control – most often hyperglycaemia, occasionally leading to metabolic decompensation.

Moreover, the incidence of sudden death is higher in patients with diabetes. Compared with non-diabetic patients, there is evidence from the Global Utilization of Streptokinase and Tissue plasminogen activator for Occluded coronary arteries (GUSTO) investigators that patients with diabetes present around 15 minutes after MI.[212]

Consider an electrocardiogram if a patient presents with such symptoms. Ischaemic electrocardiograms are more commonly found in asymptomatic diabetic patients than in non-diabetics. There is some evidence from observational studies that abnormalities of the QT interval may have prognostic implications in patients with diabetes; several studies have confirmed an independent relation between prolonged QT interval duration, or increased QT interval dispersion, and CAD.[213]

> *Acute myocardial infarction may present with atypical symptoms in diabetic patients*

Management of acute myocardial infarction in the patient with diabetes

There is no evidence that accepted therapeutic interventions are less efficacious in patients with diabetes. The acute effect of aspirin is similar in diabetics and non-diabetics. Because of their higher absolute risk, diabetics may derive even greater benefit from interventions such as thrombolysis and β-blockers. However, there is evidence that these life-preserving drugs continue to be underused in these high-risk patients.

Therefore, in addition to measures such as analgesia this should include, as appropriate:

- Aspirin – chewed at presentation and in the long-term (if there are no contraindications [300 mg at presentation and 75–150 mg thereafter])

> *The benefits of thrombolysis and β-blockers are greater in diabetic patients reflecting their higher absolute risk*

- Thrombolysis – the benefits of prompt thrombolysis are at least as great in patients with diabetes. Some patients with diabetes are denied thrombolysis for fear of precipitating sight-threatening retinal bleeding, but this risk has been greatly overstated. Primary angioplasty may have advantages but is less widely available
- ACE inhibitors – these are indicated primarily for cardiac failure or impaired left ventricular function on echocardiogram. ARBs are increasingly regarded as alternatives for patients who develop cough. The results of recent clinical trials (see above) have led to the view that all eligible patients with CAD should receive an agent that blocks the renin–angiotensin system. However, a recent trial showed no benefit of combining therapy with an ARB and an ACE inhibitor;[214] combining valsartan with captopril increased the rate of adverse events without improving survival
- β-blockers – subgroup analyses suggest that these agents are particularly beneficial in diabetic patients. Recent trials have shown the benefits of certain drugs in the management of chronic heart failure
- Insulin–glucose infusion – with continuation of subcutaneous insulin where possible; the rationale for this approach has already been discussed
- Lipid lowering therapy – statins, started before discharge from hospital. As already discussed, recent evidence favours intensive statin therapy in the highest risk groups; patients with diabetes and coronary disease fall into this category. There is evidence of benefit emerging by 30 days.

66*The small risk of intraocular haemorrhage from retinopathy should not deter the use of thrombolysis in patients with diabetes* **99**

Revascularization procedures

In general, revascularization procedures, i.e. angioplasty and coronary artery bypass grafting, have appeared to be less effective in diabetic patients; lower patient and graft survival rates have been reported in diabetic subgroups of clinical studies. The complex pathophysiology of coronary lesions allied to multisystem dysfunction, for example abnormalities of endothelial function, platelet function and clotting in diabetic patients (see sections on *Diabetes and cardiovascular disease: an intimate relationship* and *Cardiovascular risk factors in the patient with diabetes*) contribute to inferior outcomes. However, the studies were performed in the 1980s and 1990s. With the development of drug-eluting intracoronary stents, the relative efficacy of coronary artery bypass grafting and optimal stenting procedures in conjunction with newer antiplatelet drugs is now less clear. This is a rapidly evolving area which is the subject of ongoing clinical trials.

Encouraging results for patients with diabetes have emerged from the Munich registry. Intensive therapy, using multiple advanced therapeutic strategies in diabetic patients with acute MI, has resulted in a substantial reduction in hospital mortality. Rates of hospital mortality comparable with those of non-diabetic patients have recently been reported using this approach, which included greater use of glucose–insulin infusions and stents.

Antiplatelet therapy

Platelets from patients with diabetes often have hypersensitivity in vitro to platelet-aggregating agents. A major mechanism is increased production of thromboxane, a potent vasoconstrictor that causes platelet aggregation. There is some evidence of excess thromboxane release in patients with type 2 diabetes with CVD. Aspirin blocks thromboxane synthesis by acetylating platelet cyclo-oxygenase.

- **Secondary prevention trials** – a meta-analysis of 145 prospective controlled trials of antiplatelet therapy in men and women after MI, stroke or transient ischaemic attack, or positive cardiovascular history (vascular surgery, angioplasty, angina, etc) has been reported by the Anti-Platelet Trialists' Collaboration.[215] Reductions in vascular events were about one-quarter in each of these categories, and diabetic patients had risk reductions that were comparable to non-diabetic patients. There was a trend towards increased risk reductions with doses of aspirin between 75 and 162 mg/day.
- **Primary prevention trials** – two studies have examined the effect of aspirin in primary prevention and have included patients with diabetes. The US Physicians' Health Study[216] was a primary prevention trial in which a low-dose aspirin regimen (325 mg every other day) was compared with placebo in male physicians. There was a 44% risk reduction in the treated group, and subgroup analyses in the diabetic physicians revealed a reduction in MI from 10.1% (placebo) to 4.0% (aspirin), yielding a relative risk of 0.39 for the diabetic men on aspirin therapy.

These results are supported by the Early Treatment Diabetic Retinopathy Study, a mixed primary and secondary prevention trial.[217] This population consisted of type 1 and type 2 diabetic men and women, about 48% of whom had a history of CVD. The study, therefore, may be viewed as a mixed primary and secondary prevention trial. The relative risk for MI in the first five years in those randomized to aspirin therapy was lowered significantly to 0.72 (confidence interval 0.55–0.95).

The ADA recommends aspirin therapy (75–162 mg/day) as a secondary prevention strategy in men and women with diabetes who have a history of MI, vascular bypass, stroke or TIA, peripheral vascular disease or angina.[218] For primary prevention, aspirin therapy (75–162 mg/day) is recommended in patients with type 2 diabetes at increased cardiovascular risk. The optimal dose of aspirin in diabetes is uncertain and current advice is that this should be the same as for the general population. Aspirin is used increasingly in primary prevention in high-risk patients >30 years with diabetes.[219]

In HOT,[192] half of the 18,790 patients were randomized to receive aspirin in addition to their antihypertensive medication, and half were randomized to receive placebo. The use of aspirin resulted in a 15% reduction in major cardiovascular events (8.9:10.5/1000 patient-years; p = 0.03) and a 36% reduction in MI (2.3:3.6/1000 patient-years; p = 0.002). No differences were observed between patients with or without diabetes.

For patients who have undergone insertion of coronary stents, a combination of clopidogrel and aspirin may be optimal; these agents increase platelet inhibition through synergistic mechanisms.[220]

Heart failure

Heart failure is common in patients with diabetes, especially after MI when it is a major cause of death.[221] The Framingham Heart Study showed heart failure to be twice as common in men and five times as common in women with diabetes compared with non-diabetics.[222] The association with diabetes was even stronger for patients aged 65 years or older. In the DIGAMI study (see above), heart failure was the principal cause of death in the first year after MI in patients with diabetes.[223]

Part of this risk may be mediated via obesity, which is an important risk factor for diabetes independent of other classic risk factors.[224] Patients with heart failure, whether diabetic or not, often have whole body insulin resistance.[30] Recent studies have shown that the myocardium of patients with type 2 diabetes is resistant to the action of insulin on glucose transport proportionately to insulin resistance in skeletal muscle.[153] Increased reliance on fatty acids increases myocardial oxygen consumption.

Women with type 2 diabetes reportedly have greater increases in left ventricular mass than do men, independent of age, BMI and blood pressure.[225] In the UKPDS, the prevalence of heart failure rose with elevations of glycated haemoglobin concentrations, no threshold being apparent.[137] A diabetic cardiomyopathy, with microvascular and fibrotic components, has been proposed that may help to explain the high rates of heart failure in patients with diabetes.[221] Other factors that often contribute to initiation and exacerbation of heart failure include:

- CAD
- Hypertension
- Activation of the sympathetic nervous system
- Overactivity of the renin–angiotensin system.

Left ventricular dysfunction often remains undiagnosed, and untreated, until an advanced stage – perhaps largely a reflection of the asymptomatic nature of early heart failure. The diagnosis relies on a high index of clinical suspicion allied to:

- Electrocardiography – useful for detecting ischaemia, rhythm disturbances (such as atrial fibrillation) and left ventricular hypertrophy
- Chest X-ray – may confirm cardiomegaly; lung fields may be clear in early left ventricular failure
- Cardiac ultrasound – more sensitive than electrocardiography for detecting chamber hypertrophy, and other structural changes and aspects of cardiac function. Doppler echocardiography is useful in the diagnosis of diastolic heart failure; systolic function, by definition, is preserved[226]
- Atrial natiuretic peptides – these peptides are increasingly recognized to be useful markers of subclinical and clinical heart failure.[227] A recent study suggests that elevated B-type atrial natriuretic peptide concentrations predict cardiac event and all-cause mortality in patients with type 2 diabetes.[228]

There are concerns about the use of thiazolidinediones in patients with heart failure; precautions are necessary, particularly if these drugs are combined with insulin (see section on *Thiazolidinediones*). Heart failure is more prevalent among insulin-treated patients with type 2 diabetes, reflecting longer duration of diabetes and multiple risk factors.

> *Patients with diabetes and heart failure benefit from ACE inhibitors and beta-blockers at least as much as those without diabetes*

Drug therapy

Using β-blockers and ACE inhibitors, or ARBs, prevents cardiac remodelling and declining ventricular function.[229] Treatment options include the following.

- ACE inhibitors – many trials have demonstrated the effectiveness of ACE inhibitors in heart failure in the general population. A number of these have contained significant numbers of patients with diabetes. ARBs are widely regarded as alternatives. The Candesartan in Heart failure Assessment of Reduction in Mortality and morbidity (CHARM) programme of trials[230,231]confirmed the use of this agent as an alternative to ACE inhibitors if the latter are not tolerated or contraindicated because of angioedema. However, in another study the combination of two agents from these classes, captopril and valsartan, respectively, did not improve survival but increased the rate of adverse events. Valsartan was as effective as captopril in patients at high risk for cardiovascular events after MI.[214]

- Diuretics – loop diuretics are usually needed. Risks include volume depletion with prerenal failure and hypokalaemia. There are no clinical trials of survival with these agents.
- Spironolactone – careful use in conjunction with other measures can extend survival. Care is needed in patients at risk of hyperkalaemia. Eplerenone is a recently introduced aldosterone antagonist that appears to avoid the side effects associated with spironolactone such as gynaecomastia.[232]
- β-blockers – the use of these drugs in patients with chronic stable heart failure is now well established, producing significant benefits in terms of mortality. These large clinical trials contained significant numbers of patients with diabetes who showed benefit similar to that observed in all participants.[233] β-blockers should be considered in patients with diabetes and with New York Heart Association grade II, III or IV heart failure, who are stable on combined ACE inhibitor and diuretic treatment and have no contraindications to therapy. Evidence so far supports any of bisoprolol, slow-release metoprolol or carvedilol. Treatment should be started at low doses and gradually titrated up, as tolerated, to those used in the clinical trials.
- Digoxin – this is used primarily to control ventricular rate in patients with atrial fibrillation.
- Glycaemic control – this may play a role in the therapy of heart failure in the patient with diabetes. The adverse metabolic side effects that have been associated with β-adrenergic inhibitors in the diabetic patient may be circumvented by the use of so-called third-generation β-blockers.[221]

Cerebrovascular disease

Transient hyperglycaemia may be observed after acute stroke even in the absence of a prior history of diabetes.[234] Observational studies suggest that hyperglycaemia, with stroke, at presentation is an independent marker of adverse clinical outcome with increased mortality, higher morbidity, longer hospital stays, impaired long-term recovery and reduced ability to return to work.[235]

The benefits of antihypertensive therapy in preventing cerebrovascular disease among patients with type 2 diabetes was amply demonstrated in the UKPDS – evidence that is supported by other clinical trials (see section on *High blood pressure*). Statins are also useful for reducing the risk of thromboembolic stroke (see section on *Statins*). There is evidence

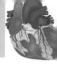

that abnormalities in coagulation and fibrinolysis may contribute to stroke.[236]

Disturbances of insulin and glucose metabolism have been implicated in Alzheimer's disease (see below).[237]

Transient focal cerebral dysfunction associated with metabolic emergencies in patients with diabetes may occasionally cause diagnostic difficulties.

- Hypoglycaemia – severe insulin- or, much less commonly, sulphonylurea-induced hypoglycaemia may resemble stroke; typical clinical features of adrenergic activation, for example, tachycardia, sweating, pallor, etc are not always present in patients with hypoglycaemia, particularly if episodes are recurrent. This phenomenon, which is associated with type 1 diabetes of long duration, is known as hypoglycaemia-associated autonomic failure.[238] Repeated episodes of severe hypoglycaemia may cause cognitive impairment. Rarely, insulin-treated patients may report transient hemiplegia on waking from sleep in the apparent absence of obvious cerebrovascular disease.

- Metabolic decompensation – the presentation of an unconscious patient with type 2 diabetes who has developed hyperosmolar non-ketotic hyperglycaemia may resemble a devastating stroke; in addition, transient focal neurological signs may accompany marked hyperglycaemia. A bedside capillary blood test will readily reveal marked hyperglycaemia.

- Seizures – generalized tonic-clonic epileptic convulsions can result from either severe acute hypo- or hyperglycaemia. Therefore, blood glucose concentration should be measured in any patient presenting with symptoms or signs suggestive of stroke.

- Cognitive function in older adults – diabetes and impaired fasting glucose are associated with impaired cognitive performance.[239] An interaction between diabetes and apolipoprotein E genotypes has been reported.[240] At the cellular level, diabetes increases brain amyloid deposition and neurofibrillary tangles. Associated defects, notably hyperinsulinaemia, have been associated with a higher risk of Alzheimer's disease and decline in memory.[241] Other vascular risk factors such as dietary fat intake, blood lipids and hypertension may conspire with hyperglycaemia to increase the risk of both vascular and Alzheimer's dementia.[242]

Animal studies have shown that raising blood glucose levels acutely can help memory, in part, by increasing cholinergic activity, which is markedly diminished in patients with Alzheimer's disease. Other studies have confirmed that glucose administration can help memory in healthy humans and in patients with Alzheimer's disease. Therefore, the picture is complex.[237]

"Severe hypo- and hyperglycaemia may be associated with acute neurological deficits"

Management

Careful attention to risk factor modification is essential to prevent primary and recurrent events. A multidisciplinary approach to management is required to optimize outcome. For acute events, this is best undertaken during the acute phase and during early rehabilitation in specialist stroke units.

> **In patients with atrial fibrillation and diabetes, anticoagulation with warfarin should be considered where there are no contra-indications**

*   Hypertension – tight control of hypertension reduces the risk of stroke in patients with type 2 diabetes.[191] There has been debate about whether certain agents, either as monotherapy or in combination, offer advantages. Overall, blood pressure reduction reduces stroke by around 30–40%. Achieving the target blood pressure appears to be more important than the choice of drugs.[243]

*   Antiplatelet therapy – aspirin 50–350 mg daily is recommended for most patients with type 2 diabetes to prevent thrombotic stroke and other cardiovascular events. It is prudent to ensure that blood pressure is controlled (systolic <150 mmHg) before initiating aspirin therapy as primary preventive therapy. Options to reduce the risk of recurrent ischaemic stroke include combination low-dose aspirin 25 mg + dipyridamole 200 mg b.d. or clopidogrel 75 mg in the case of aspirin allergy.[244] The role of thrombolysis for selected patients with acute ischaemic stroke is less well defined, and practice varies widely between countries.

*   Statins – recent statin studies have shown a welcome reduction in thromboembolic stroke. Allocation to simvastatin 40 mg daily in the Heart Protection Study reduced the rate of ischaemic strokes by about one-quarter. However, after making allowance for non-compliance in the trial, this regimen would probably reduce the stroke rate by about one-third.[245] This was true regardless of the pre-treatment LDL level or whether CAD was present. The aforementioned CARDS, for example, documented a 48% reduction in thrombotic stroke in patients with type 2 diabetes.[167] Some authorities suggest that such benefit is greater than would be predicted from the epidemiological evidence linking LDL cholesterol with stroke.

> **In patients with diabetes, atherosclerosis has a predilection for vessels below the popliteal fossa**

*   Warfarin – because of the high risk of stroke in patients with diabetes and atrial fibrillation,[32] anticoagulation with warfarin should be considered as a primary prevention measure against thromboembolic stroke, where no contraindications exist and where benefits of therapy are thought to outweigh risks of haemorrhage. Serious co-morbidity among patients with diabetes, for example advanced renal failure or uncontrolled hypertension, may adversely alter the risk–benefit equation.

*   Carotid endarterectomy – careful selection of symptomatic patients and timely surgery is needed;[246] patients with asymptomatic lesions

or those who have had TIAs or an ipsilateral non-disabling thromboembolic stroke are potentially candidates for this procedure.

Peripheral arterial disease

Although the incidence of PAD is increased among diabetic patients,
accurate data are hard to obtain. A recent population-based survey
suggests that PAD affects more than 5 million US adults.[247] The
prevalence increases dramatically with age and disproportionately
affects black people.

The risk of peripheral arterial disease is increased among patients with diabetes

In concert with neuropathy and infection, PAD contributes to foot
disease in patients with diabetes. Among classic risk factors, arterial
hypertension, smoking and dyslipidaemia are associated with increased
risk of peripheral arterial disease.[247] In the UKPDS, each 1% increase
in glycated haemoglobin was associated with a 28% increased risk of
PAD, and each 10 mmHg increase in systolic blood pressure conferred
a 25% increase in risk.[248]

Compromise of arterial supply leads to secondary defects in intracellular metabolism with the development of a complex metabolic
myopathy.[249]

Atherosclerosis in the leg of the patient with diabetes has a
predilection for vessels below the popliteal fossa. The explanation for
this distal distribution has not been adequately explained. Symptoms,
which depend on the site and degree of the stenosis, may include:

- Intermittent claudication – classic calf claudication on walking;
  neuropathy may modify or attenuate symptoms in patients with
  diabetes. This is the usual presenting feature of aorto-ilio-femoral
  atherosclerosis. More subtle impairment of functional capacity is
  also common

Peripheral arterial disease usually indicates the presence of atherosclerosis on other arterial beds

- Rest pain – denotes critical ischaemia with high risk of limb loss;
  usually distal disease. Critical ischaemia is associated with a high
  short-term case fatality rate
- Leriche syndrome – buttock and leg claudication, with erectile
  dysfunction due to major stenosis of the aorto-femoral vessels
- Ischaemic foot lesions – ischaemia alone probably accounts for
  <10% of diabetes-related foot ulcers. However, arterial ischaemia is
  a significant contributor in neuro-ischaemic lesions, which com-
  prise around 50% of all foot ulcers among patients with diabetes.
  Ischaemic ulceration tends to affect areas such as the medial and
  lateral aspects of the foot and the heel. In contrast to neuropathic
  ulcers, which usually develop over high-pressure areas such as the
  first metatarsal head, an arterial ulcer is often painful. Ischaemic
  ulcers are not usually associated with the formation of callus
- PAD is indicative of a high risk of other CVD, notably CAD.[33]

Table 23. Ratio of the ankle pressure (the highest of readings from the dorsalis pedis and posterior tibial arteries) to the brachial artery pressure (the highest from both arms). Note: poorly compressible vessel if >1.30 interpretation of ankle–brachial pressure index. Data from American Diabetes Association. Peripheral arterial disease in people with diabetes. *Diabetes Care* 2003;26:3333–3341.

Normal	0.91–1.30
Mild disease	0.70–0.90
Moderate disease	0.40–0.69
Severe disease	<0.40

Therefore, the discovery of peripheral arterial disease should prompt a thorough review of cardiovascular risk factors.

Assessing the peripheral vasculature

The annual review of adults with diabetes should include an assessment of the peripheral arterial system.

- Physical examination – this should include manual palpation of all the peripheral pulses and auscultation for bruits. The absence of dorsalis pedis and posterior tibial arteries, when assessed by an experienced observer, is regarded as a reliable indicator of peripheral arterial disease. Around 10% of non-diabetic patients have an absent pedal pulse, the posterior tibial artery being the pulse most consistently present. Trophic changes in the skin are sought. The limb is pale and cold in the presence of significant ischaemia, but may have a reddish hue with critical impairment of blood flow, the so-called sunset foot. Buerger's sign may be positive: the limb blanches on being raised above the horizontal plane, subsequently assuming a dusky-red colour when placed in a dependent position.
- Treadmill test – a graded treadmill test may aid diagnosis and permit assessment of functional capacity and response to treatment.
- Doppler studies – these are readily performed by trained personnel at the bedside using a handheld Doppler probe.[250] Doppler studies are recommended in all patients with diabetes who have absent pedal pulses or foot ulceration. The ratio of the ankle pressure (the highest of readings from the dorsalis pedis and posterior tibial arteries) to the brachial artery pressure (the highest from both arms) is normally around 1.0–1.3 (Table 23). The ratio may be falsely elevated by medial arterial calcification that is often present in patients with diabetes of long duration; the calcification renders the vessels resistant to compression by the ankle pressure cuff. The quality of the Doppler signal may be informative. Normally, three components can be discerned, i.e. the signal is said to be 'triphasic'. With arterial calcification there may be a biphasic or monophasic signal. Further assessment may then be indicated. Patients with symptomatic claudication usually have a drop in ankle pressure of >20 mmHg after exercise.

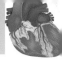

Specialist investigations

- Duplex scanning – this useful, non-invasive technique combines ultrasound imaging with Doppler assessment of blood flow to provide information about the haemodynamic significance of lesions. However, calcification may limit the quality of the information obtained. Duplex scanning is usually a prelude to angiography if surgery is contemplated.
- Oxygen tension – this can be measured transcutaneously on the dorsum of the foot using a laser Doppler probe allowing confirmation of critical ischaemia. A partial pressure of <30 mmHg is held to predict poor wound healing.
- Arterial angiography – this investigation delineates the site and extent of the lesions, which often affect the distal arterial tree. Magnetic resonance angiography is a non-invasive alternative that is less widely available. Care should be taken to ensure adequate hydration in patients with nephropathy undergoing imaging with iodinated contrast agents. Note that serum creatinine concentrations may be misleadingly satisfactory in patients, particularly elderly women, in the presence of significant renal dysfunction. This reflects low skeletal muscle mass, from which creatinine is derived. Calculated creatinine clearance is a better way to determine risk. Temporary withdrawal of metformin (see section on *Metformin*) may be prudent because temporary renal impairment due to contrast nephropathy may lead to accumulation of the drug with a risk of lactic acidosis.

Medical management

Treatment should be two-fold: (1) primary and secondary cardiovascular risk factor modification and (2) treatment of symptoms, i.e. claudication and critical limb ischemia, allied to limiting the progression of disease. In fact, there is little in the way of prospective data specifically in patients with peripheral arterial disease and diabetes showing that treating risk factors improves cardiovascular outcomes. With this proviso in mind, there have been a number of advances in the medical management of peripheral arterial disease in recent years.[33]

- Tobacco avoidance – this is regarded as essential to prevent progression of atheroma with risk of amputation. Smoking is one of the most important modifiable risk factors for peripheral arterial disease. Cessation counselling should be available to all patients. Pharmacological modulation of the endocannabinoid system is under evaluation (see above).
- Anti-platelet agents – aspirin reduces mortality from CVD in patients with diabetes and is recommended where there are no

contraindications. However, the Antiplatelet Trialists' Collaboration showed no significant reduction in deaths among a subgroup of patients with claudication.[215] Clinical trial evidence supporting use of clopidogrel in patients with diabetes and peripheral arterial disease is more convincing, the reduction in vascular events being superior to aspirin in the Clopidogrel versus Aspirin in Patients at Risk of Ischaemic Events (CAPRIE) study; this evaluated aspirin versus clopidogrel in more than 19,000 patients with recent stroke, MI or stable peripheral arterial disease.[251]

- A daily dose of 75 mg of clopidogrel was associated with a relative risk reduction of 8.7%, compared with the benefits of 325 mg of aspirin per day for a composite end point (MI, ischaemic stroke and vascular death). In a subgroup analysis of more than 6000 patients with peripheral arterial disease, clopidogrel was associated with a risk reduction of 24%, compared with aspirin. Around one-third of the patients in the latter group had diabetes. In those patients, clopidogrel was also superior to aspirin therapy. Clopidogrel was as well tolerated as aspirin.

- Lipid-lowering therapy – should be considered in all patients because they are usually at very high risk of macrovascular events in all major territories: statins are the drugs of choice. In the HPS, simvastatin produced a marginally significant reduction in the number of participants who developed peripheral macrovascular complications.[163]

- Treatment of high blood pressure – hypertension is a major risk factor for CVD and this is regarded as a logical reason to treat high blood pressure in patients with PAD. Note the risks arising from renal artery stenosis and caution with ACE inhibitors and ARBs in patients with peripheral arterial disease, and potential adverse effects of β-blockers on claudication.

- Glycaemic control – more intensive treatment of hyperglycaemia did not reduce the incidence of peripheral arterial disease among middle-aged patients with type 2 diabetes in the UKPDS.[129] Nonetheless, diabetes is a risk factor for critical limb ischaemia.[252] Identification and treatment of diabetes is regarded as an important aspect of the prevention of cardiovascular events in general.[253]

- Foot care – patients should receive appropriate instruction. Regular inspection by a trained professional and timely podiatry may avert the development of more serious lesions.

- Supervised exercise programmes – by improving the collateral circulation, these can improve walking distance over several months; unsupervised exercise prescriptions are largely ineffective. At least three months of intermittent treadmill walking three times per week is needed.

- Ginkgo biloba – there is evidence for some efficacy.
- Pentoxifylline – the mechanism of action of this drug, which is approved for use by the US Food and Drug Administration, is uncertain. The dose is 400 mg t.d.s. with meals. The dose should be reduced in patients with cirrhosis. Pain-free walking distance is improved.
- Cilotazol – this recently introduced oral phosphodiesterase type 3 inhibitor is a vasodilator that can increase pain-free walking distance; the drug is US Food and Drug Administration approved. Use is contraindicated in patients with heart failure or low cardiac ejection fraction.[254]

Invasive interventions

Reconstructive surgery, or angioplasty in selected cases, may preserve limbs. Two major patterns are seen, which carry different prospects for successful intervention:
- Proximal disease – patients with weak femoral pulses and absent distal pulses may be suitable for angioplasty or arterial bypass grafting. Localized short stenoses are most suitable for angioplasty
- Distal disease – this is more common in diabetes and is much more difficult to treat by angioplasty or bypass grafting.

In subintimal angioplasty a controlled dissection is created; it is a minimally invasive procedure that can be used to recanalize long occluded segments of arteries. Amputation should be avoided wherever possible, but is sometimes the only option. Major amputation is associated with an appreciable short-term mortality.

The challenge of multifactorial risk management

66The cardiovascular risk conferred by hypertension and dyslipidaemia in combination is at least additive 99

Clinical trials in diabetes have generally focused on the effectiveness of single interventions, and few data are available concerning simultaneous treatment of multiple risk factors. The effects of a target-driven, intensified intervention aimed at multiple risk factors in patients with type 2 diabetes compared with usual care has recently been reported.[136]

In the previously mentioned Steno-2 study, 160 patients with type 2 diabetes and microalbuminuria were randomized to either intensive treatment using ACE inhibitors and aspirin (blood pressure control target 130/80 mmHg, haemoglobin A1c <6.5%, total cholesterol <4.5mmol/l, triglycerides <1.7mmol/l) or conventional treatment (blood pressure target 135/85 mmHg, haemoglobin A1c 6.5%, total cholesterol <4.9 mmol/l, triglycerides <2 mmol/l) and aspirin only for manifest CAD.

"Multiple risk factor intervention reduces vascular events in patients with diabetes"

Over a mean follow up of 7.8 years, blood pressure, serum cholesterol, serum triglycerides and haemoglobin A_{1c} were significantly lower in the intensive-treated group, compared with the conventionally treated group. Associated with these improvements, there was a highly significant reduction in the risk of any cardiovascular event, including MI, from 44% to 24% with intensive treatment. Concomitant reductions in nephropathy, retinopathy and autonomic neuropathy were also seen (Figure 29). This approach was of benefit to both microvascular and macrovascular complications; increasingly clinicians must endeavour to ensure that both aspects of the vasculopathy of diabetes are addressed.

The role of the diabetes health care team

Having established the effectiveness of multiple interventions in diabetes, major challenges remain in ensuring that appropriate patients are targeted. Issues such as long-term compliance with increasingly complex drug regimens represent formidable obstacles. In pursuit of best practice, diabetes educators, clinical nurse specialists, dietitians and podiatrists all have potential, and currently underappreciated, roles.[25,255] The frequency of patient contact that is often needed by these professionals offers opportunities for reinforcing the principles of cardiovascular risk reduction.

Moreover, members of professions allied to medicine may be better placed than the supervising clinician to glean insights into day-to-day barriers to effective therapy for individual patients. Appropriate education of relevant healthcare professionals is needed, including that for neglected groups such as nursing home staff. Efficient sharing of clinical and laboratory data between those involved in the delivery of diabetes health care is another important, and currently underdeveloped, consideration.

Figure 29. Panel A. Mean changes in selected risk factors in the intensive-therapy group and the conventional-therapy group during follow up. Panel B. Percentage of patients in each group who reached the intensive-treatment goals at a mean of 7.8 years. In panel A mean annual values are shown for the patients in the intensive-therapy group, whereas mean values obtained at the three examinations – at baseline, after four years, and after eight years – are shown for the conventional-therapy group. (LDL = low-density lipoprotein; BP = blood pressure. To convert values for cholesterol to mmol/l, multiply by 0.02586; to convert values for triglycerides to mmol/l, multiply by 0.01129). Reproduced with permission from *N Engl J Med* 2003;348:383–393. Copyright © 2003 Massachusetts Medical Society. All rights reserved.

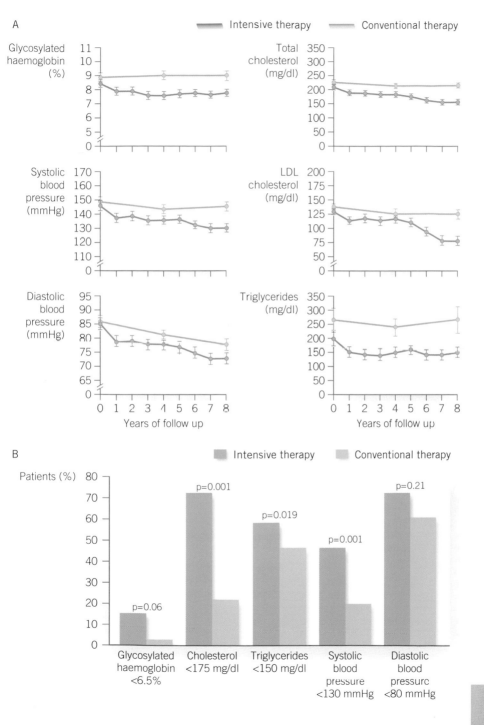

Future prospects

Observational data from the USA provide some encouragement that the risk of CVD among patients with diabetes has reduced during recent decades.[256] However, rapidly increasing rates of obesity and the metabolic syndrome at ever younger ages threaten to reverse this trend in dramatic fashion.

For those who develop CVD, the results of the recent multicentre DIGAMI 2 study indicate that with modern management, mortality rates after MI among patients with diabetes can approach those of non-diabetics.[151] Evidence of the importance of intensive glycaemic control, in concert with other measures, to clinical outcomes in selected high-risk patients is steadily accumulating.[257]

However, action at population level will also be necessary if we are to counter the challenges posed by diabetes and the metabolic syndrome in the twenty-first century.

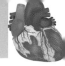

CASE STUDIES

Case study 1

Silent myocardial infarction in a patient with type 2 diabetes

Mr A is a 58-year-old warehouse supervisor, who was found to have gly-cosuria at a routine examination at work nine years ago. A fasting blood glucose was 16.3 mmol/l and hyperglycaemia was confirmed by a sub-sequent measurement. At the time he was overweight with a BMI of 28.6 kg/m^2; his blood pressure was 120/88 mmHg. Peripheral pulses were palpable and his fundi were normal on ophthalmoscopy. His calo-rie intake – including a reported three pints of beer a day – was esti-mated to be around 3000 calories. He is a non-smoker.

Relevant biochemical investigations include:

• Glycated haemoglobin (HbA$_{1c}$)	10.0%	High
• Total cholesterol	3.1 mmol/l	Normal
• HDL cholesterol	1.2 mmol/l	Normal
• Fasting triglycerides	2.4 mmol/l	High
• Creatinine	90 µmol/l	normal

12-lead electrocardiogram (ECG) was normal.

(Note: reference ranges may differ between laboratories.)

Comment and management

Mr A was advised to start a diet of 1800 calories per day and to increase his habitual level of physical activity. In the absence of contraindica-tions, such as renal impairment, he was also started on metformin 500 mg t.d.s. This drug was shown in the UKPDS 34 trial to be effective in reducing cardiac mortality in overweight newly diagnosed patients with type 2 diabetes randomized to the drug as monotherapy.

One of the main pieces of advice was to reduce markedly his beer intake. Mr A is a bachelor and enjoys playing snooker, an activity that in his case is closely associated with beer drinking!

Because Mr A's total cholesterol concentration was regarded as being satisfactory, no lipid-lowering medication was prescribed. It was noted that his triglycerides were raised, but it was hoped that the level would improve as his diabetes came under control.

Over the last decade, clinical trials – particularly involving statins – have indicated that a statin might be started at this point, the aim

It was hoped that his triglyceride level would improve as his diabetes came under control

being to reduce Mr A's global cardiovascular risk. In this context, diabetes has come to be regarded as a 'coronary risk equivalent' deserving of statin therapy. The HPS trial demonstrated benefits of simvastatin 40 mg in patients with diabetes. More recently, the CARDS trial showed significant benefits from atorvastatin 10 mg in patients with type 2 diabetes. Therefore, the concept of a 'normal' cholesterol level is somewhat erroneous in the presence of other major risk factors.

Progress

At review six months later Mr A had lost 6 kg in weight and his HbA_{1c} had fallen to a satisfactory level of 4.9%. This improvement was attributed in part to a decrease in his alcohol intake, allied to other changes in diet and the actions of metformin. Unfortunately, he regained 4 kg in weight over the following year.

The following year he developed ulceration of his second toe, which subsequently healed with conservative measures. He continued to maintain good glycaemic and blood pressure control.

Four years ago he became concerned about episodes of tightness in his chest, not always related to exertion. A repeat ECG suggested an old inferior infarct. He was started on atenolol 25 mg daily. This is an effective drug for cardioprotection post MI, particularly in diabetic patients, and the advantages in such cases outweigh any drug-induced impairment of insulin sensitivity. β-blockers are effective anti-anginal drugs. An exercise ECG revealed no reversible ischaemic changes.

Atenolol is an effective drug for cardioprotection post MI

Atorvastatin 10 mg was also added, lowering his total cholesterol to 2.8 mmol/l, raising his HDL cholesterol to 1.4 mmol/l and reducing his triglycerides to 2.0 mmol/l. Aspirin 75 mg was added to reduce the risk of arterial thrombosis.

Two years ago he was noted to have background retinopathy and required additional medication to keep his HbA_{1c} below 7%: rosiglitazone 4 mg daily was added. A thiazolidinedione was felt to be preferable to a sulphonylurea drug. Certain sulphonylureas have adverse effects on ischaemic preconditioning, although the clinical significance of this effect remains uncertain.

Sulphonylureas have long been added to metformin, although a cloud was cast over this combination in the UKPDS trial, a finding that caused some concern at the time. Thiazolidinediones may have beneficial cardiovascular effects beyond glucose lowering, which are currently under scrutiny in clinical trials. Therefore, the choice of a thiazolidinedione reflects the promise of theoretical cardiovascular benefits. Mr A's blood pressure remains well controlled at 120/65 mmHg.

Thiazolidinediones may have beneficial cardiovascular effects beyond glucose lowering

Learning points

- Diabetes substantially increases the risk of myocardial infarction. The latter may present atypically – clinically silent infarcts are well recognized.
- This patient developed coronary disease despite apparently good control of his glucose levels and having levels of cholesterol and blood pressure that were regarded as satisfactory. His non-smoking status helped to protect him against the development of cardiovascular disease. Use of drugs such as statins reduces cardiovascular events in diabetes but does not completely eliminate the risk. Recent trials suggest that aggressive lowering of LDL cholesterol may be advantageous to patients at the highest levels of risk, a category that includes patients who have diabetes accompanied by cardiovascular disease. LDL cholesterol may be calculated from the Friedewald formula; this is regarded as reliable in the absence of marked hypertriglyceridaemia and is often reported by clinical chemistry laboratories.
- It is now widely thought to be appropriate to offer most middle-aged patients with diabetes a statin to reduce global risk unless contraindicated. Strict targets for patients with cardiovascular disease may require high-dose statins or consideration of combination therapy with the cholesterol-absorption inhibitor ezetimibe (although clinical outcome data are not available for this combination). Control of triglycerides and raising low levels of HDL cholesterol are increasingly regarded as secondary targets requiring separate measures, such as consideration of a fibrate (take care in combination with statins because there is an increased risk of serious myositis) or nicotinic acid. When fasting triglycerides exceed approximately 1.5–2.0 mmol/l, atherogenic small, dense LDL cholesterol particles tend to predominate (although they cannot be measured using routine laboratory methods).

"This patient developed coronary disease despite apparently good control of his glucose levels and having satisfactory levels of cholesterol and blood pressure"

Type 2 diabetes in an active, non-obese elderly patient

Mr M is an 80-year-old, active, retired, successful businessman. Relevant conditions include well-controlled hypertension of 130/80 mmHg and a history of gout for which he takes allopurinol. His diabetes was diagnosed when he complained of fatigue and thirst; a random blood glucose was 17.5 mmol/l. He was taking atenolol 50 mg daily and doxazosin 1 mg daily, thiazides having been stopped after he developed gout.

An attempt to change his β-blocker to an ACE inhibitor resulted in a dry cough, a common side effect of the latter class; he was then switched to an angiotensin receptor blocker. However, he requested to go back on his β-blocker because he was more confident with it, his GP's reluctance notwithstanding.

He was drinking two bottles of wine per week and was a non-smoker. No vascular complications were evident on physical examination. His BMI was normal at 23 kg/m^2.

Relevant biochemical investigations include:		
• HbA$_{1c}$	8.5%	High
• Total cholesterol	3.6 mmol/l	Normal
• HDL cholesterol	1.1 mmol/l	Low–normal
• Fasting triglycerides	2.1 mmol/l	High
• Urea	5.5 mmol/l	Normal
• Creatinine	107 µmol/l	Normal

Comment and management

The diagnosis is type 2 diabetes in an active elderly man with a 20-year history of essential hypertension and no apparent vascular complications. Dietary advice was deemed appropriate to see whether reduction of simple sugars and alcohol intake could control his blood sugar levels, but in fact his HbA$_{1c}$ three months later was unsatisfactory at 8.5% and his lipid pattern was unchanged. Apart from his glass and a half of wine at night, his diet appeared to be healthy.

Mr M was therefore started on metformin 500 mg, one tablet a day for the first fortnight, increasing to one tablet twice daily for the second fortnight and then finally increased to the present dose of 500 mg three times a day. The gradual introduction was to minimize the

"Dietary advice was deemed appropriate to see whether reduction of simple sugars and alcohol could control his blood sugar levels"

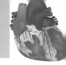

potential gastrointestinal disturbances often associated with the drug. Simvastatin 10 mg daily and aspirin 75 mg daily were also prescribed.

Progress

Two years on Mr M is leading a full and active life. His latest HbA_{1c} is excellent (5.8%) and his total cholesterol has declined to 3.0 mmol/l. His triglycerides have also reduced to a healthier level of 1.4 mmol/l. He shows no diabetic complications.

Learning points

- Even in the elderly diabetes should be actively treated, as long as treatment does not impair quality of life unduly. Symptoms can usually be controlled and the risk of vascular complications reduced. Many elderly patients will ultimately require insulin – usually after combinations of oral antidiabetic agents have been tried – and often cope remarkably well. Age *per se* should not preclude the use of optimal therapy.
- The trend in diabetes is an increasing tendency to so-called polypharmacy, driven by evidence from clinical trials. Patients need to be warned that optimal management may necessitate taking a number of drugs. Avoiding drugs with side effects and use of once-daily formulations aid compliance; many patients do not derive the benefits of medication through non-concordance with their prescribed regimen. Combinations of drugs, e.g. ACE inhibitor plus diuretic, calcium channel blocker with statin, are increasingly being introduced. Long scorned by clinical pharmacologists such preparations may also aid long-term compliance.
- Polypharmacy in the elderly carries greater risks of adverse drug reactions. These may arise because of drug–drug interactions or because of the development of long-term tissue complications. Note that renal impairment is a contraindication to metformin therapy. Careful periodic monitoring is therefore necessary because renal impairment is common.
- The dose of simvastatin used in the HPS trial was 40 mg daily. This dose would be appropriate in the light of the efficacy demonstrated in this trial.

❝Patients need to be warned that optimal management may necessitate taking a number of drugs ❞

Case study 3
Attaining therapeutic targets in the face of psychological problems

Mr C is a 51-year-old, non-smoking teacher, off work with stress-related psychological problems. He sought advice about an axillary furuncle; urinalysis revealed glycosuria. He is sent for blood tests, which confirm diabetes. His blood pressure is 160/100 mmHg and his BMI is 42 kg/m².

Relevant biochemical investigations include:		
• Fasting glucose	17.0 mmol/l	High
• HbA$_{1c}$	9.8%	High
• Urea	3.4 mmol/l	Normal
• Creatinine	70 µmol/l	Normal
• Total cholesterol	5.4 mmol/l	Normal
• HDL cholesterol	1.7 mmol/l	Normal
• Fasting triglycerides	2.0 mmol/l	High

Eye examination revealed normal fundi.

Comment and management

The target blood pressure for Mr C is 130/80 mmHg and the target HbA$_{1c}$ is <7%. He has morbid obesity so needs advice from a dietitian. His LDL cholesterol is elevated at 3.7 mmol/l but nonetheless would benefit from a reduction.

Mr C is started on an ACE inhibitor, lisinopril, which is gradually increased in dosage, and metformin was chosen for blood glucose control because he is obese (UKPDS 34). Simvastatin 10 mg is introduced to lower his cholesterol and lipid levels along with aspirin 75 mg daily.

His normal fundi are reassuring, but steps should be taken to minimize the risk of developing retinopathy.

His normal fundi are reassuring but steps should be taken to minimize the risk of developing retinopathy

Progress

Mr C's mental health deteriorated and on the advice of a psychiatrist he was started on haloperidol 1 mg twice daily. Despite possible adverse metabolic effects of this drug (an issue recently highlighted with so-called atypical agents), his blood glucose has remained under good control on metformin 500 mg t.d.s, even though his BMI has increased to 44 kg/m². His total cholesterol has reduced to 4.6 mmol/l and triglycerides to 1.2 mmol/l.

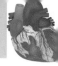

However, his blood pressure has been more stubborn, probably not being helped by his increasing weight. The lisinopril was titrated up to 20 mg daily and then bendrofluazide, a thiazide diuretic, was added in at a dose of 2.5 mg daily. A β-blocker was also added in the hope that this might have a beneficial effect on his anxiety, but he developed erectile dysfunction with this, so a calcium channel blocker (felodipine) was substituted and titrated up to 10 mg daily.

Finally, doxazosin was added at a dose of 4 mg daily. With quadruple therapy his blood pressure (assuming compliance) is currently 135/85 mmHg.

Learning points

- With strict blood pressure targets difficult to attain, triple and quadruple therapy is often necessary. In general, use low doses of each agent to minimize the potential for adverse effects; consider combination preparations.
- Moxonidine can be a useful add-in drug and might be used if his blood pressure rises again in the future; check for contraindications to the use of this centrally acting sympatholytic agent.
- Control of blood pressure is highly desirable and complements the vascular protection attained through improved long-term glycaemic control (UKPDS 38 and 39).
- With his psychiatric problems it was very difficult to motivate Mr C to lose weight or take exercise, although walking would be beneficial for both his weight and mental problems. Depression is very common among patients with type 2 diabetes and presents additional hurdles to management. More serious psychiatric conditions, e.g. schizophrenia, are associated with an increased risk of diabetes and cardiovascular disease, and are thought to be mediated at least in part by unhealthy lifestyles.

❝In general, use low doses of each agent to minimize the potential for adverse effects❞

Case study 4
Non-compliant patient with type 2 diabetes

He subsequently ignored advice about treatment for around 10 years

Mr D is a 40-year-old brewery worker and heavy drinker (an occupational hazard!) who was found to have glycosuria when he presented to the genitourinary clinic with balanitis. He was diagnosed with diabetes on the basis of a fasting glucose measurement.

He subsequently ignored advice about treatment for around 10 years until he attended his doctor with pain in the scapular region. His BMI was 30 kg/m^2 and blood pressure 160/95 mmHg. He was persuaded to have some further blood tests.

Relevant biochemical investigations include:

• HbA$_{1c}$	12.8%	High
• Fasting glucose	16.9 mmol/l	High
• Total cholesterol	8.6 mmol/l	High
• HDL cholesterol	1.0 mmol/l	Normal
• Urea	7.4 mmol/l	High
• Creatinine	99 µmol/l	Normal
• Urinary albumin dipstick	++	High
• Gamma glutamyl transferase	144 IU/l	High
Other liver function tests were normal.		

Comment and management

Mr D has all the features of poorly controlled diabetes and the metabolic syndrome. Added to this he has significant hypercholesterolaemia. Eight pints a day of beer is contributing to his poor health. He has a slightly raised urea and a normal creatinine, suggesting that his kidney function may be starting to deteriorate and hinting towards what will ensue. Because he was feeling well and was reluctant to modify his lifestyle he continued to ignore medical advice.

His kidney function may be starting to deteriorate hinting towards what will ensue

Progress

Some 18 years after being originally diagnosed as having diabetes Mr D attended his GP because he had erectile dysfunction. After the GP explained the condition and its consequences Mr D agreed to accept treatment for his diabetes.

He was started on metformin, simvastatin and lisinopril. An ACE inhibitor was chosen because this is most appropriate for his hypertension in the presence of proteinuria; this most likely indicates diabetic nephropathy. His erectile dysfunction did not respond to sildenafil. A second oral antidiabetic agent was added in, in the form of gliclazide, a sulphonylurea. Further antihypertensive agents were also added, the calcium channel blocker amlodipine and then the β-blocker doxazosin.

Mr D was found to have significant microvascular complications: he had sight-threatening retinopathy, painful peripheral neuropathy in his feet, and a raised urea of 11.1 mmol/l with a creatinine that had risen to 119 µmol/l. He was offered laser therapy for his retinopathy but initially refused when told that it is not always successful. Soon after, he had a vitreous haemorrhage so was persuaded to reconsider. Four years later and after bilateral cataract operations, he had 6/9 sight in both eyes with only a slight amount of field loss in his left eye.

Subsequently he was admitted to hospital following an episode of severe hypoglycaemia. The metformin and gliclazide were stopped because his urea had risen to 21.6 mmol/l and his creatinine to 300 µmol/l. His HbA$_{1c}$, while not taking any anti-diabetic drugs, remained apparently satisfactory at 6.2% (but see below) and his total cholesterol was 3.7 mmol/l.

He is now under the care of the renal unit and has been told that his renal function is likely to continue to deteriorate and that he may need dialysis. Good control of his diabetes and, more importantly at this stage, his blood pressure should help to retard progression to end-stage renal failure. In fact, his blood pressure (128/65 mmHg) is good on the following medication:

- Doxazosin 8 mg daily
- Moxonidine 400 µg daily
- Amlodipine 10 mg daily
- Perindopril 8 mg daily.

He is also receiving:

- Simvastatin 20 mg daily
- Calcium resonium 15 g on alternate days (anion-exchange resin for hyperkalaemia).

Erythropoietin therapy is due to be started for his nephropathy-associated anaemia, his haemoglobin being reduced at 10.4 g/dl.

"An ACE inhibitor was chosen because this is most appropriate for his hypertension in the presence of proteinuria"

121

Learning points

- This man continued in his job with its associated heavy drinking lifestyle for 20 years before his loss of vision as a result of vitreous haemorrhage brought compliance. With appropriate treatment his vision was saved.

- He was not so lucky with his kidney function and dialysis now looks inevitable.

- The case illustrates why metformin is contraindicated in the presence of renal failure: the drug is excreted unchanged via the kidney. The drug accumulates increasing the risk of hypoglycaemia (when combined with a sulphonylurea) and exposing the patient to the risk of lactic acidosis. Sulphonylureas should be used with considerable caution at this level of renal impairment, if at all. The risk of severe hypoglycaemia may be increased by heavy alcohol consumption. Short-acting insulin releasing drugs, e.g. repaglinide, may be safer, but insulin is often the best option for patients not controlled by diet alone. Note that anaemia, present in this case, will cause a false low HbA_{1c} result: his glycaemic control may not be as good as it appears. Random glucose levels should be also be measured.

- ACE inhibitors and angiotensin receptor blockers slow the rate of decline of renal function in patients with type 2 diabetes. Care should be taken to re-check the serum creatinine within one or two weeks of starting these drugs because bilateral renal artery stenosis may lead to a precipitous decline in renal function. Watch for hyperkalaemia in patients on potassium-sparing drugs in the presence of renal impairment.

- Statins are generally safe in patients with renal impairment and should be used whenever possible to reduce the greatly magnified risk of cardiovascular disease that accompanies renal failure. Many patients with type 2 diabetes who develop nephropathy will succumb to myocardial infarction before needing renal replacement therapy. Fibrates should be avoided in patients with renal failure.

> *Note that anaemia will cause a false low HbA_{1c} result*

> *Many patients with nephropathy will succumb to myocardial infarction before needing renal replacement therapy*

Case study 5

The metabolic syndrome – and more: a recipe for cardiovascular disease

Mr L has a strong family history of both premature heart disease and type 2 diabetes. His father died at age 62 from a myocardial infarction and his father's first infarct occurred when he was 52. His uncle died suddenly of a heart attack at age 59. His personal medical history includes obstructive sleep apnoea. He quit smoking 20 years ago. His alcohol intake is reportedly 28 units per week. His BMI is 44 kg/m^2 and blood pressure 120/90 mmHg (confirmed by retesting using a large cuff).

Five years ago the following results were noted:

• Total cholesterol	5.6 mmol/l	Normal
• HDL cholesterol	1.07 mmol/l	Low–normal
• Fasting glucose	6.3 mmol/l	High
• 2-hour serum glucose (after 75 g challenge)	10.2 mmol/l	High
• Fasting triglycerides	5.9 mmol/l	High
• HbA$_{1c}$	5.2%	Normal

Comment and management

The clinical chemistry results show that Mr L had morbid obesity with marked hypertriglyceridaemia. His fasting glucose was raised. In the absence of additional data he would fall into the category of impaired fasting glucose. A 75 g oral glucose tolerance test confirmed that he did not have diabetes at this point, the 2-hour level being diagnostic of impaired glucose tolerance. Diastolic hypertension was also present as judged by current diagnostic criteria for the metabolic syndrome.

He was referred to the lipid clinic and lost 9 kg of weight in the first four weeks on a calorie-restricted diet. He then regained 2 kg the following month and did not return to the clinic after that point for follow-up measurements of his triglycerides. Atenolol was started, as much for a complaint of palpitations as for his raised diastolic blood pressure: his blood pressure was lowered to 120/80 mmHg and his palpitations resolved.

Two years later he was diagnosed as having diabetes when he turned up at the surgery with excessive thirst; a random blood glucose was unequivocally elevated at 25.6 mmol/l. He was started on metformin and additional blood tests were requested.

The results were:		
• Total cholesterol	7.9 mmol/l	High
• Triglycerides	31.9 mmol/l	Very high
• HbA$_{1c}$	10.9%	High

The biochemist phoned Mr L's GP to warn of the greatly raised triglycerides with their risk of acute pancreatitis. Mr L was started on simvastatin, but developed what was thought to be an allergic rash; a similar problem occurred with metformin, although such reactions are rare with either drug. Indeed, a diabetologist stated that this was the first case of metformin allergy he had seen or heard of, but was seemingly convinced by the evidence before him. Intolerance of a drug – whether real or perceived – inevitably engenders reluctance to persevere with the therapy.

"Mr L realized he faced a stark choice – his job or his long-term health "

Progress

Mr L was able to follow dietary advice, losing 16 kg over eight weeks. He reduced his alcohol consumption and started taking regular walks. His blood pressure improved to 102/68 mmHg while taking atenolol 25 mg daily. His triglycerides fell to 4.5 mmol/l and his cholesterol to 4.6 mmol/l, without pharmaceutical intervention. Subsequently, fenofibrate 267 mg daily was added and his triglycerides declined to 3.2 mmol/l. However, he lost his job and took another that involved working long hours in another betting shop too far from home for him to walk to. He found himself unable to comply with diet and exercise advice and his weight shot up, his BMI rising to 46 kg/m². Rosiglitazone was added because glycaemic control had deteriorated.

Mr L realized he faced a stark choice – his job or his long-term health. He resigned from the bookmakers, and is now walking his dog three miles a day. Once again he is losing weight and is back down to a BMI of 44 kg/m².

Learning points

- Mr L has a combination of obesity, hypertriglyceridaemia, glucose intolerance and diastolic hypertension. He satisfies all of the main criteria for the metabolic syndrome, as defined by the National Cholesterol Education Program 2001. Added to this he has a disturbing family history of premature coronary disease and has sleep apnoea, regarded as a facet of the spectrum of chronic disorders associated with insulin resistance. Developing diabetes added still further to his global risk of cardiovascular disease. There can be little doubt that he falls into a very high category of risk for atherosclerosis.

- He developed a very high level of triglycerides, which put him at risk of pancreatitis but exercise, diet and weight loss helped reverse this. Genetic factors may be operating. A low-fat diet is an important aspect of management. Fibrates are often effective and are the lipid-lowering drugs of choice. Statins generally have only modest effects on triglyceride levels. For patients with diabetes insulin can also sometimes be very effective for controlling major hypertriglyceridaemia.

- Without time to exercise sufficiently or to eat regular, healthy meals he is struggling to lose weight. The chances of major weight loss in patients with morbid obesity, other than surgically induced, are remote. Nonetheless, modest weight loss can improve adverse cardiovascular risk profiles. Moreover, the benefits of regular exercise in reducing risk may be somewhat underestimated.

- Did the β-blocker accelerate the progression to diabetes (and possibly aggravate his dyslipidaemia?). This cannot be determined, but current advice from the British Hypertension Society cautions against the use of agents from this class, and in particular the combination with thiazide diuretics, in such circumstances. It is recognized that many β-blockers promote weight gain, aggravate lipid disturbances and exacerbate insulin resistance. Unless there is a pressing indication, e.g. angina, alternative agents with more favourable metabolic profiles should be used. ACE inhibitors, angiotensin receptor blockers, calcium antagonists, moxonidine and α-blockers are more suitable.

- Rosiglitazone will not help his obesity but may improve several aspects of the metabolic syndrome. However, this drug seems to be less consistent in lowering triglycerides than pioglitazone. Both drugs improve HDL cholesterol levels, but the impact on cardiovascular events is presently uncertain. Eagerly awaited clinical trial results are expected in the latter half of 2005.

"He satisfies all of the main criteria for the metabolic syndrome"

"The chances of major weight loss in patients with morbid obesity, other than surgically induced, are remote"

"Did the beta-blocker accelerate the progression to diabetes?"

APPENDIX 1: DRUGS USED TO TREAT DIABETES

Sulphonylureas

Generic name	Trade names	Daily dose	Duration of action*	Main route of elimination	Main unwanted effects	Other comments
First generation					By stimulating insulin secretion all sulphonylureas have the capacity to cause hypoglycaemia, which may occasionally be severe. Longer-acting agents such as glibenclamide carry the highest risk. Care is required in the elderly, the infirm and patients with renal impairment	
Chlorpropamide	Generic	100–500mg	Long	Urine >90%		Requires adequate endogenous insulin secretion
Tolbutamide‡	Generic	500–2000mg	Short	Urine ~100%		Always start with the lowest dose and gradually increase towards the maximum in stages every few weeks
Second generation						
Glibenclamide§	Daonil, Semi-Daonil, Euglucon	2.5–15mg	Intermediate to long	Bile ~50%		Maximal glucose-lowering effects are usually obtained at doses lower than the manufacturer's recommendations
Gliclazide	Diamicron	40–320mg#	Intermediate	Urine ~65%		Effects of sulphonylureas on vascular function depend on presence or absence of benzamido group; glimepiride and gliclazide reportedly are largely devoid of the adverse effects on ischaemic preconditioning that have been demonstrated experimentally with glibenclamide
Glimepiride	Amaryl	1–6mg	Intermediate	Urine ~80%		
Glipizide†	Glibenese, Minodiab	2.5–20mg	Short to intermediate	Urine ~70%		
Gliquidone	Glurenorm	15–180mg	Short to intermediate	Bile ~95%	Weight gain of ~1–4 kg is common	

Not all of these preparations are available in every country.

* Long >24 hours; intermediate 12–24 hours; short <12 hours.

‡ Should be taken immediately before meals.

§ Glibenclamide is known as glyburide in the USA. In the USA, a micronized formulation of glibenclamide is available that increases the rate of gastrointestinal absorption, thereby enabling an earlier onset of action.

† A longer-acting (extended release) formulation of glipizide has also been introduced in the USA.

Modified (extended) release preparation, Diamicron MR dose range 30–120 mg. Gliclazide is not available in the USA.

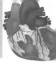

Rapid-acting secretagogues

Generic name	Trade names	Daily dose	Duration of action*	Main route of elimination	Main unwanted effects	Other comments
Nateglinide	Starlix	60–120mg immediately before main meals	Short‡	Hepatic	Hypoglycaemia, although this risk is generally lower than for the sulphonylureas	Rapid-acting insulin releasers must be timed to coincide with the main meal. If a meal is skipped, the relevant dose of repaglinide is omitted
Repaglinide	NovoNorm	0.5–4mg immediately before each main meal to a maximum of 16mg daily	Short‡	Hepatic	Weight gain: this also tends to be less marked than with sulphonylureas	Repaglinide may be a useful alternative to sulphonylureas in patients with erratic meal patterns or mild to moderate renal impairment

In the UK nateglinide is licensed for use only in combination with metformin |

* Long >24 hours; intermediate 12–24 hours; short <12 hours.
‡ Main effect is in the immediate post-prandial period ~3 hours.

127

Biguanides

Generic name	Trade names	Daily dose	Duration of action*	Main route of elimination	Main unwanted effects	Other comments
Metformin	Glucophage	500–2500mg in divided doses‡	Short$	Renal	Gastrointestinal symptoms may limit compliance Risk of lactic acidosis in certain clinical situations	Start with 500mg daily and slowly increase dose Avoid in patients with renal impairment, cardiac decompensation or acute coronary syndromes; discontinue temporarily if contrast imaging studies are performed Often used in combination with other agents, most commonly sulphonylureas or thiazolidinediones

Metformin is the only preparation available in the UK and USA.

* Long >24 hours; intermediate 12–24 hours; short <12 hours.

‡ 3000mg in some countries.

$ An extended release formulation – Glucophage SR – is available in some countries.

Combination preparations, e.g. Glucovance (glibenclamide + metformin) and Avandamet (rosiglitazone + metformin) have become available in recent years.

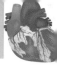

Alpha-glucosidase inhibitors

Generic name	Trade names	Daily dose	Duration of action*	Main route of elimination	Main unwanted effects	Other comments
Acarbose	Glucobay	50–150mg daily in divided doses	Short‡	The small amount of intestirally generated degradation products that are absorbed are eliminated renally	Gastrointestinal side effects: flatus and abdominal pain predominate	Avoid in patients with intestinal disorders The glucose-lowering effect of acarbose is relatively modest May be combined with drugs from other classes

* Long >24 hours; intermediate 12–24 hours; short <12 hours.
‡ Acarbose reduces post-prandial hyperglycaemia; little effect on fasting glucose levels.
Miglitol and voglibose are also available in some countries.

Thiazolidinediones

Generic name	Trade names	Daily dose	Duration of action*	Main route of elimination	Main unwanted effects	Other comments
Pioglitazone	Actos	15–45mg daily‡	Intermediate$	Bile	Weight gain of ~5% is common	Glucose-lowering effect requires several weeks to become maximal
Rosiglitazone	Avandia	2–8mg daily‡	Intermediate$	Urine	Oedema may develop in ~5%; concerns about potential for precipitating heart failure is greatest in patients on combination therapy with insulin; use in conjunction with insulin is contraindicated in some countries	Avoid in patients with heart failure – details vary between countries Do not use in patients with active liver disease; for monitoring of liver function tests consult local licensing details

* Long >24 hours; intermediate 12–24 hours; short <12 hours.

‡ Licences and dosages vary between countries and according to whether used as monotherapy or in combination with other agents, e.g. sulphonylureas.

$ Glucose-lowering effect may persist for some time after discontinuation of therapy.

Insulin preparations

Category	Generic name	Trade name	Onset of action*	Duration of action*
Rapid	Insulin aspart Insulin lispro	NovoRapid Humalog	10–20 minutes 10 minutes	3–4 hours 10–20 hours
Rapid–intermediate	Biphasic insulin aspart Biphasic insulin lispro	NovoMix 30 Humalog Mix 25 Humalog Mix 50	10 minutes	10–20 hours
Short	Soluble	Actrapid Humulin S Insuman Rapid	15–60 minutes	4–8 hours
Short–intermediate	Biphasic isophane insulin	Humulin M3 Insuman Comb Mixtard	15–60 minutes	12–20 hours
Intermediate	Isophane NPH insulin	Insulatard Humulin I	60–120 minutes	12–20 hours
Long	Insulin zinc suspension (crystalline) Insulin detemir Insulin glargine	Ultratard Humulin Zn Levemir Lantus	120–240 minutes 60–120 minutes	18–24 hours 18–24 hours

* Times of onset and duration of action are approximate ranges that vary between individuals, with dose and site of subcutaneous injection and pathophysiological state. NPH = neutral protamine Hagedorn.

APPENDIX 2: ABBREVIATIONS

Abbreviations	
General	
ACE	Angiotensin converting enzyme
ADA	American Diabetes Association
AGE	Advanced glycation end products
AIDS	Acquired immune deficiency syndrome
ARB	Angiotensin receptor blocker
BHS	British Hypertension Society
BMI	Body mass index
CAD	Coronary artery disease
CVD	Cardiovascular disease
ECG	Electrocardiogram
HbA_{1c}	Glycated haemoglobin
HDL	High-density lipoprotein
HRT	Hormone replacement therapy
IDL	Intermediate-density lipoprotein
IGF-1	Insulin-like growth factor-1
IGT	Impaired glucose tolerance
LDL	Low-density lipoprotein
MI	Myocardial infarction
NAFLD	Non-alcoholic fatty liver disease
NCEP	National Cholesterol Education Program
NICE	National Institute for Clinical Excellence
PAD	Peripheral arterial disease
PCOS	Polycystic ovary syndrome
PPAR	Peroxisome proliferator-activated receptor
TIA	Transient ischaemic attack
TNF-α	Tumour necrosis factor-α
VCAM-1	Vascular cell adhesion molecule-1
VLDL	Very-low-density lipoprotein
WHO	World Health Organization

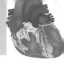

Clinical trials

4S	Scandinavian Simvastatin Survival Study
ALLHAT	Antihypertensive and Lipid-Lowering treatment to Prevent Heart Attack Trial
ASCOT-LLA	Anglo-Scandinavian Cardiac Outcomes Trial-Lipid Lowering Arm
BARI 2D	Bypass Angioplasty Revascularization Investigation in type 2 Diabetes
CAPRIE	Clopidogrel versus Aspirin in Patients at Risk of Ischaemic Events
CARDS	Collaborative Atorvastatin Diabetes Study
CARE	Cholesterol and Recurrent Events
CHARM	Candesartan in Heart failure Assessment of Reduction in Mortality and morbidity
DAIS	Diabetes Atherosclerosis Intervention Study
DCCT	Diabetes Control and Complications Trial
DECODE	Diabetes Epidemiology: Collaborative analysis of Diagnostic criteria in Europe
DIGAMI	Diabetes Mellitus and Insulin–Glucose Infusion in Acute Myocardial Infarction
DPP	Diabetes Prevention Program
DREAM	Diabetes REduction Assessment with ramipril and rosiglitazone Medication
EPIC	European Prospective Investigation into Cancer and nutrition
EUROPA	EUROpean trial on reduction of cardiac events with Perindopril in stable coronary Artery disease
GUSTO	Global Utilization of Streptokinase and Tissue plasminogen activator for Occluded coronary arteries
HDS	Hypertension in Diabetes Study
HERS	Heart and Estrogen/progestin Replacement Study
HOPE	Heart Outcomes Prevention Evaluation
HOT	Hypertension Optimal Treatment
HPS	Heart Protection Study
LIFE	Losartan Intervention For Endpoint in hypertension
MIRACL	Myocardial Ischemia Reduction with Aggressive Cholesterol Lowering
NAVIGATOR	Nateglinide and Valsartan in Impaired Glucose Tolerance Outcomes Research

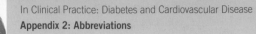

Clinical trials

ONTARGET	ONgoing Telmisartan Alone and in combination with Ramipril Global Endpoint Trial
PEACE	Prevention of Events with Angiotensin Converting Enzyme inhibitor trial
PROactive	Prospective Pioglitazone Clinical Trial in Macrovascular Events
PROVE-IT	Pravastatin or Atorvastatin Evaluation and Infection Therapy–Thrombolysis in Myocardial Infarction Study
RECORD	Rosiglitazone Evaluated for Cardiac Outcomes and Regulation of glycaemia in Diabetes
SHEP	Systolic Hypertension in the Elderly Program
STOP-NIDDM	Study TO Prevent Non-Insulin Dependent Diabetes Mellitus
SYST-EUR	Systolic Hypertension-Europe
UGDP	University Group Diabetes Program
UKPDS	United Kingdom Prospective Diabetes Study
VA-HIT	Veterans Administration High density lipoprotein Intervention Trial
WHI	Women's Health Initiative

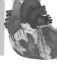

APPENDIX 3: WEBSITES FOR USEFUL ORGANIZATIONS

American Association of Clinical Endocrinologists
www.aace.com

American Association of Diabetes Educators
www.aadenet.org

American College of Cardiology
www.acc.org

American Diabetes Association
www.diabetes.org

American Heart Association
www.americanheart.org

British Heart Foundation
www.bhf.org.uk

British Hypertension Society
www.bhsoc.org

Diabetes Australia
www.diabetesaustralia.com.au

Diabetes UK
www.diabetes.org.uk

European Association for the Study of Diabetes
www.easd.org

European Group for the Study of Insulin Resistance
www.egir.org

International Diabetes Federation
www.idf.org

International Society of Diabetes and Vascular Disease
www.intsocdvd.com

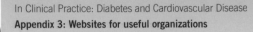

Juvenile Diabetes Research Foundation International
www.jdf.org

National Institute of Diabetes and Digestive and Kidney Diseases
www.niddk.nih.gov

Society for Endocrinology
www.endocrinology.org

World Health Organization
www.who.int

APPENDIX 4: REFERENCES

1. Beckman JA, Creager MA, Libby P. Diabetes and atherosclerosis: epidemiology, pathophysiology, and management. *JAMA* 2002;287:2570–81.

2. Yusuf S, Hawken S, Ounpuu S et al. Effect of potentially modifiable risk factors associated with myocardial infarction in 52 countries (the INTERHEART study): case-control study. *Lancet* 2004;364:937–52.

3. Wild S, Roglic G, Green A et al. Global prevalence of diabetes: estimates for the year 2000 and projections for 2030. *Diabetes Care* 2004;27:1047–53.

4. Gu K, Cowie CC, Harris MI. Diabetes and decline in heart disease mortality in US adults. *JAMA* 1999;281:1291–7.

5. Kopelman PG. Obesity as a medical problem. *Nature* 2000;404: 635–43.

6. Mokdad AH, Bowman BA, Ford ES et al. The continuing epidemics of obesity and diabetes in the United States. *JAMA* 2001;286:1195–200.

7. Grundy SM. Obesity, metabolic syndrome, and cardiovascular disease. *J Clin Endocrinol Metab* 2004;89:2595–600.

8. Cooper R, Cutler J, Desvigne-Nickens P et al. Trends and disparities in coronary heart disease, stroke, and other cardiovascular diseases in the United States: findings of the national conference on cardiovascular disease prevention. *Circulation* 2000;102:3137–47.

9. Engelgau MM, Geiss LS, Saaddine JB et al. The evolving diabetes burden in the United States. *Ann Intern Med* 2004;140:945–50.

10. Ten S, Maclaren N. Insulin resistance syndrome in children. *J Clin Endocrinol Metab* 2004;89:2526–39.

11. Barrett-Connor EL, Cohn BA, Wingard DL et al. Why is diabetes mellitus a stronger risk factor for fatal ischemic heart disease in women than in men? The Rancho Bernardo Study. *JAMA* 1991;265:627–31.

12. Barrett-Connor E, Giardina EG, Gitt AK et al. Women and heart disease: the role of diabetes and hyperglycemia. *Arch Intern Med* 2004;164:934–42.

13. Kanaya AM, Grady D, Barrett-Connor E. Explaining the sex difference in coronary heart disease mortality among patients with type 2 diabetes mellitus: a meta-analysis. *Arch Intern Med* 2002;162:1737–45.

14. Barrett-Connor E, Ferrara A. Isolated postchallenge hyperglycemia and the risk of fatal cardiovascular disease in older women and men. The Rancho Bernardo Study. *Diabetes Care* 1998;21:1236–9.

15. Hu FB, Stampfer MJ, Haffner SM et al. Elevated risk of

cardiovascular disease prior to clinical diagnosis of type 2 diabetes. *Diabetes Care* 2002;25:1129–34.

16. Wilson PWF. Epidemiology of hyperglycemia and atherosclerosis. In: Ruderman N, Williamson J, Brownlee M (eds). Hyperglycemia, diabetes and vascular disease. New York: Oxford University Press, 1992:21–9.

17. Langer RD. Hormone replacement and the prevention of cardiovascular disease. *Am J Cardiol* 2002;89:36E–46E; discussion 46E.

18. Stork S, van der Schouw YT, Grobbee DE et al. Estrogen, inflammation and cardiovascular risk in women: a critical appraisal. *Trends Endocrinol Metab* 2004;15:66–72.

19. Hulley S, Grady D, Bush T et al. Randomized trial of estrogen plus progestin for secondary prevention of coronary heart disease in postmenopausal women. Heart and Estrogen/progestin Replacement Study (HERS) Research Group. *JAMA* 1998;280:605–13.

20. Women's Health Initiative Investigators. Risks and benefits of estrogen plus progestin in healthy postmenopausal women. Heart and Estrogen/progestin Replacement Study. *JAMA* 2002;288:321–33.

21. Barrett-Connor E. Clinical review 162: cardiovascular endocrinology 3: an epidemiologist looks at hormones and heart disease in women. *J Clin Endocrinol Metab* 2003;88:4031–42.

22. Raza JA, Reinhart RA, Movahed A. Ischemic heart disease in women and the role of hormone therapy. *Int J Cardiol* 2004;96:7–19.

23. Executive Summary of The Third Report of The National Cholesterol Education Program (NCEP) Expert Panel on Detection, Evaluation, And Treatment of High Blood Cholesterol In Adults (Adult Treatment Panel III). *JAMA* 2001;285:2486–97.

24. Haffner SM, Lehto S, Ronnemaa T et al. Mortality from coronary heart disease in subjects with type 2 diabetes and in nondiabetic subjects with and without prior myocardial infarction. *N Engl J Med* 1998;339:229–34.

25. Williams B, Poulter NR, Brown MJ et al. Guidelines for management of hypertension: report of the fourth working party of the British Hypertension Society, 2004-BHS IV. *J Hum Hypertens* 2004;18:139–85.

26. Aguilar D, Solomon SD, Kober L et al. Newly diagnosed and previously known diabetes mellitus and 1-year outcomes of acute myocardial infarction: the VALsartan In Acute myocardial iNfarcTion (VALIANT) trial. *Circulation* 2004;110:1572–8.

27. Garg A. Statins for all patients with type 2 diabetes: not so soon. *Lancet* 2004;364:641–2.

28. Stevens RJ, Kothari V, Adler AI et al. The UKPDS risk engine: a model for the risk of coronary heart disease in Type II diabetes (UKPDS 56). *Clin Sci (Lond)* 2001;101:671–9.

29. Bell DS. Diabetic cardiomyopathy. *Diabetes Care* 2003;26:2949–51.

30. Doehner W, Anker SD, Coats AJ. Defects in insulin action in chronic heart failure. *Diabetes Obes Metab* 2000;2:203–12.

31. Amato L, Paolisso G, Cacciatore F et al. Congestive heart failure predicts the development of non-insulin-dependent diabetes mellitus in the elderly. The Osservatorio Geriatrico Regione Campania Group. *Diabetes Metab* 1997;23:213–18.

32. Davis TM, Millns H, Stratton IM et al. Risk factors for stroke in type 2 diabetes mellitus: United Kingdom Prospective Diabetes Study (UKPDS) 29. *Arch Intern Med* 1999;159:1097–103.

33. Krentz AJ, Shearman CP. Peripheral arterial disease and diabetes: time for action. *Br J Diab Cardiovasc Dis* 2003;3:92–6.

34. Stamler J, Vaccaro O, Neaton JD et al. Diabetes, other risk factors, and 12-yr cardiovascular mortality for men screened in the Multiple Risk Factor Intervention Trial. *Diabetes Care* 1993;16:434–44.

35. Kannel WB, D'Agostino RB, Sullivan L et al. Concept and usefulness of cardiovascular risk profiles. *Am Heart J* 2004;148:16–26.

36. Reaven G. The metabolic syndrome or the insulin resistance syndrome? Different names, different concepts, and different goals. *Endocrinol Metab Clin North Am* 2004;33:283–303.

37. Haffner SM, Stern MP, Hazuda HP et al. Cardiovascular risk factors in confirmed prediabetic individuals. Does the clock for coronary heart disease start ticking before the onset of clinical diabetes? *JAMA* 1990;263:2893–8.

38. Haffner SM, Mykkanen L, Festa A et al. Insulin-resistant prediabetic subjects have more atherogenic risk factors than insulin-sensitive prediabetic subjects: implications for preventing coronary heart disease during the prediabetic state. *Circulation* 2000;101:975–80.

39. Reaven GM. Banting lecture 1988. Role of insulin resistance in human disease. *Diabetes* 1988;37:1595–607.

40. Meigs JB. The metabolic syndrome. *BMJ* 2003;327:61–2.

41. Sun H, Kim GMR. The metabolic syndrome: one step forward, two steps back. *Diabetes Vasc Dis Res* 2004;1:68–75.

42. Alberti KG, Zimmet PZ. Definition, diagnosis and classification of diabetes mellitus and its complications. Part 1: diagnosis and classification of diabetes mellitus provisional report of a WHO consultation. *Diabet Med* 1998;15:539–53.

43. World Health Organization. Definition, diagnosis and classification of diabetes mellitus and its complications: reports of a WHO consultation. Part 1: diagnosis and classification of diabetes mellitus.

139

Geneva: World Health Organization, 1998.

44. Balkau B, Charles MA. Comment on the provisional report from the WHO consultation. European Group for the Study of Insulin Resistance (EGIR). *Diabet Med* 1999;16:442–3.

45. Bloomgarden ZT. American Association of Clinical Endocrinologists (AACE) consensus conference on the insulin resistance syndrome: 25–26 August 2002, Washington, DC. *Diabetes Care* 2003;26:1297–303.

46. Hu G, Qiao Q, Tuomilehto J et al. Prevalence of the metabolic syndrome and its relation to all-cause and cardiovascular mortality in nondiabetic European men and women. *Arch Intern Med* 2004;164:1066–76.

47. Ford ES, Giles WH, Dietz WH. Prevalence of the metabolic syndrome among US adults: findings from the third National Health and Nutrition Examination Survey. *JAMA* 2002;287:356–9.

48. Alexander CM, Landsman PB, Teutsch SM et al. NCEP-defined metabolic syndrome, diabetes, and prevalence of coronary heart disease among NHANES III participants age 50 years and older. *Diabetes* 2003;52:1210–4.

49. Krentz AJ. Insulin resistance. *BMJ* 1996;313:1385–9.

50. Yki-Jarvinen H. Ectopic fat accumulation: an important cause of insulin resistance in humans. *J R Soc Med* 2002;95(Suppl 42): 39–45.

51. Day CP. Pathogenesis of steatohepatitis. *Best Pract Res Clin Gastroenterol* 2002;16:663–78.

52. Glueck CJ, Papanna R, Wang P et al. Incidence and treatment of metabolic syndrome in newly referred women with confirmed polycystic ovarian syndrome. *Metabolism* 2003;52:908–15.

53. Legro RS. Polycystic ovary syndrome and cardiovascular disease: a premature association? *Endocr Rev* 2003;24:302–12.

54. Lord JM, Flight IH, Norman RJ. Metformin in polycystic ovary syndrome: systematic review and meta-analysis. *BMJ* 2003;327:951–3.

55. Krentz AJ. Insulin resistance. Oxford: Blackwell Publishing, 2002.

56. Musso C, Cochran E, Moran SA et al. Clinical course of genetic diseases of the insulin receptor (type A and Rabson-Mendenhall syndromes): a 30-year prospective. *Medicine (Baltimore)* 2004;83:209–22.

57. Chandran M, Phillips SA, Ciaraldi T et al. Adiponectin: more than just another fat cell hormone? *Diabetes Care* 2003;26:2442–50.

58. Tershakovec AM, Frank I, Rader D. HIV-related lipodystrophy and related factors. *Atherosclerosis* 2004;174:1–10.

59. Hegele RA. Premature atherosclerosis associated with monogenic

insulin resistance. *Circulation* 2001;103:2225–9.

60. Neel JV. Diabetes mellitus: a "thrifty" genotype rendered detrimental by "progress"? *Am J Hum Genet* 1962;14:353–62.

61. Hales CN, Barker DJ. The thrifty phenotype hypothesis. *Br Med Bull* 2001;60:5–20.

62. Stout RW. The impact of insulin upon atherosclerosis. *Horm Metab Res* 1994;26:125–8.

63. Ruige JB, Assendelft WJ, Dekker JM et al. Insulin and risk of cardiovascular disease: a meta-analysis. *Circulation* 1998;97:996–1001.

64. Group TDIS. Plasma insulin and cardiovascular mortality in non-diabetic European men and women: a meta-analysis of data from eleven prospective studies. *Diabetes Care* 2004;47:1245–56.

65. Tamminen MK, Westerbacka J, Vehkavaara S et al. Insulin therapy improves insulin actions on glucose metabolism and aortic wave reflection in type 2 diabetic patients. *Eur J Clin Invest* 2003;33:855–60.

66. Evans A, Krentz AJ. Benefits and risks of transfer from oral agents to insulin in type 2 diabetes mellitus. *Drug Saf* 1999;21:7–22.

67. Hsueh WA, Quinones MJ. Role of endothelial dysfunction in insulin resistance. *Am J Cardiol* 2003;92:10J–17J.

68. DeFronzo RA. Pathogenesis of type 2 diabetes mellitus. *Med Clin North Am* 2004;88:787–835, ix.

69. Gerich JE. Physiology of glucose homeostasis. *Diabetes Obes Metab* 2000;2:345–50.

70. Shulman GI. Cellular mechanisms of insulin resistance. *J Clin Invest* 2000;106:171–6.

71. Vlassara H, Palace MR. Glycoxidation: the menace of diabetes and aging. *Mt Sinai J Med* 2003;70:232–41.

72. Association AD. Diagnosis and classification of diabetes mellitus. *Diabetes Care* 2004;27:S5–S10.

73. Festa A, D'Agostino R, Jr., Hanley AJ et al. Differences in insulin resistance in nondiabetic subjects with isolated impaired glucose tolerance or isolated impaired fasting glucose. *Diabetes* 2004;53:1549–55.

74. Kuusisto J, Mykkanen L, Pyorala K et al. NIDDM and its metabolic control predict coronary heart disease in elderly subjects. *Diabetes* 1994;43:960–7.

75. Turner RC, Millns H, Neil HA et al. Risk factors for coronary artery disease in non-insulin dependent diabetes mellitus: United Kingdom Prospective Diabetes Study (UKPDS: 23). *BMJ* 1998;316:823–8.

76. Gerstein HC, Yusuf S. Dysglycaemia and risk of cardiovascular

disease. *Lancet* 1996;347:949–50.

77. Khaw KT, Wareham N, Luben R et al. Glycated haemoglobin, diabetes, and mortality in men in Norfolk cohort of european prospective investigation of cancer and nutrition (EPIC–Norfolk). *BMJ* 2001;322:15–8.

78. Fuller JH, Shipley MJ, Rose G et al. Coronary-heart-disease risk and impaired glucose tolerance. The Whitehall study. *Lancet* 1980;1:1373–6.

79. Saydah SH, Loria CM, Eberhardt MS et al. Subclinical states of glucose intolerance and risk of death in the U.S. *Diabetes Care* 2001;24:447–53.

80. Qiao Q, Jousilahti P, Eriksson J et al. Predictive properties of impaired glucose tolerance for cardiovascular risk are not explained by the development of overt diabetes during follow-up. *Diabetes Care* 2003;26:2910–4.

81. Glucose tolerance and mortality: comparison of WHO and American Diabetes Association diagnostic criteria. The DECODE study group. European Diabetes Epidemiology Group. Diabetes Epidemiology: Collaborative analysis Of Diagnostic criteria in Europe. *Lancet* 1999;354:617–21.

82. Levitan EB, Song Y, Ford ES et al. Is nondiabetic hyperglycemia a risk factor for cardiovascular disease? A meta-analysis of prospective studies. *Arch Intern Med* 2004;164:2147–55.

83. Chaves PH, Kuller LH, O'Leary DH et al. Subclinical cardiovascular disease in older adults: insights from the Cardiovascular Health Study. *Am J Geriatr Cardiol* 2004;13:137–51.

84. Heine RJ, Balkau B, Ceriello A et al. What does postprandial hyperglycaemia mean? *Diabet Med* 2004;21:208–13.

85. Muntner P, He J, Chen J et al. Prevalence of non-traditional cardiovascular disease risk factors among persons with impaired fasting glucose, impaired glucose tolerance, diabetes, and the metabolic syndrome: analysis of the Third National Health and Nutrition Examination Survey (NHANES III). *Ann Epidemiol* 2004;14:686–95.

86. Chiasson JL, Josse RG, Gomis R et al. Acarbose treatment and the risk of cardiovascular disease and hypertension in patients with impaired glucose tolerance: the STOP–NIDDM trial. *JAMA* 2003;290:486–94.

87. Hanefeld M, Chiasson JL, Koehler C et al. Acarbose slows progression of intima-media thickness of the carotid arteries in subjects with impaired glucose tolerance. *Stroke* 2004;35:1073–8.

88. Krentz AJ. Type 2 diabetes and cardiovascular disease: do they share common antecedents? *Br J Diabet Vasc Dis* 2002;2:370–8.

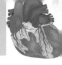

89. Singleton JR, Smith AG, Russell JW et al. Microvascular complications of impaired glucose tolerance. *Diabetes* 2003;52:2867–73.

90. Carr MC, Brunzell JD. Abdominal obesity and dyslipidemia in the metabolic syndrome: importance of type 2 diabetes and familial combined hyperlipidemia in coronary artery disease risk. *J Clin Endocrinol Metab* 2004;89:2601–7.

91. Krentz AJ. Lipoprotein abnormalities and their consequences for patients with type 2 diabetes. *Diabetes Obes Metab* 2003;5(Suppl 1):S19–27.

92. Austin MA, Hokanson JE, Edwards KL. Hypertriglyceridemia as a cardiovascular risk factor. *Am J Cardiol* 1998;81:7B–12B.

93. Ginsberg HN. Insulin resistance and cardiovascular disease. *J Clin Invest* 2000;106:453–8.

94. Barrett-Connor E, Grundy SM, Holdbrook MJ. Plasma lipids and diabetes mellitus in an adult community. *Am J Epidemiol* 1982;115:657–63.

95. Despres JP, Lamarche B, Mauriege P et al. Hyperinsulinemia as an independent risk factor for ischemic heart disease. *N Engl J Med* 1996;334:952–7.

96. Sniderman AD. Applying apoB to the diagnosis and therapy of the atherogenic dyslipoproteinemias: a clinical diagnostic algorithm. *Curr Opin Lipidol* 2004;15:433–8.

97. Lu W, Resnick HE, Jablonski KA et al. Non-HDL cholesterol as a predictor of cardiovascular disease in type 2 diabetes: the strong heart study. *Diabetes Care* 2003;26:16–23.

98. Sowers JR. Treatment of hypertension in patients with diabetes. *Arch Intern Med* 2004;164:1850–7.

99. El-Atat F, Aneja A, McFarlane S et al. Obesity and hypertension. *Endocrinol Metab Clin North Am* 2003;32:823–54.

100. Hypertension in Diabetes Study (HDS): I. Prevalence of hypertension in newly presenting type 2 diabetic patients and the association with risk factors for cardiovascular and diabetic complications. *J Hypertens* 1993;11:309–17.

101. Nesto RW. Correlation between cardiovascular disease and diabetes mellitus: current concepts. *Am J Med* 2004;116(Suppl 5A):11S–22S.

102. Reaven GM, Lithell H, Landsberg L. Hypertension and associated metabolic abnormalities—the role of insulin resistance and the sympathoadrenal system. *N Engl J Med* 1996;334:374–81.

103. Chobanian AV, Bakris GL, Black HR et al. The Seventh Report of the Joint National Committee on Prevention, Detection, Evaluation, and Treatment of High Blood Pressure: the JNC 7

report. *JAMA* 2003;289:2560–72.

104. Association AD. Nephropathy in diabetes. *Diabetes Care* 2004;27:s79–s83.

105. Hostetter TH. Chronic kidney disease predicts cardiovascular disease. *N Engl J Med* 2004;351:1344–6.

106. Kambham N, Markowitz GS, Valeri AM et al. Obesity-related glomerulopathy: an emerging epidemic. *Kidney Int* 2001;59: 1498–509.

107. Chen J, Muntner P, Hamm LL et al. The metabolic syndrome and chronic kidney disease in U.S. adults. *Ann Intern Med* 2004;140:167–74.

108. Mogensen CE. Microalbuminuria and hypertension with focus on type 1 and type 2 diabetes. *J Intern Med* 2003;254:45–66.

109. Karalliedde J, Viberti G. Microalbuminuria and cardiovascular risk. *Am J Hypertens* 2004;17:986–93.

110. Pearson TA. New tools for coronary risk assessment: what are their advantages and limitations? *Circulation* 2002;105:886–92.

111. Fonseca V, Desouza C, Asnani S et al. Nontraditional risk factors for cardiovascular disease in diabetes. *Endocr Rev* 2004;25:153–75.

112. Nesto R. C-reactive protein, its role in inflammation, Type 2 diabetes and cardiovascular disease, and the effects of insulin-sensitizing treatment with thiazolidinediones. *Diabet Med* 2004;21:810–7.

113. Ridker PM, Cushman M, Stampfer MJ et al. Inflammation, aspirin, and the risk of cardiovascular disease in apparently healthy men. *N Engl J Med* 1997;336:973–9.

114. Ridker PM, Buring JE, Shih J et al. Prospective study of C-reactive protein and the risk of future cardiovascular events among apparently healthy women. *Circulation* 1998;98:731–3.

115. Ridker PM, Buring JE, Cook NR et al. C-reactive protein, the metabolic syndrome, and risk of incident cardiovascular events: an 8-year follow-up of 14 719 initially healthy American women. *Circulation* 2003;107:391–7.

116. Malinow MR, Bostom AG, Krauss RM. Homocyst(e)ine, diet, and cardiovascular diseases: a statement for healthcare professionals from the Nutrition Committee, American Heart Association. *Circulation* 1999;99:178–82.

117. Weiss R, Dziura J, Burgert TS et al. Obesity and the metabolic syndrome in children and adolescents. *N Engl J Med* 2004;350:2362–74.

118. Tounian P, Aggoun Y, Dubern B et al. Presence of increased stiffness of the common carotid artery and endothelial

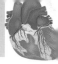

dysfunction in severely obese children: a prospective study. *Lancet* 2001;358:1400–4.

119. Saydah SH, Fradkin J, Cowie CC. Poor control of risk factors for vascular disease among adults with previously diagnosed diabetes. *JAMA* 2004;291:335–42.

120. Tuomilehto J, Lindstrom J, Eriksson JG et al. Prevention of type 2 diabetes mellitus by changes in lifestyle among subjects with impaired glucose tolerance. *N Engl J Med* 2001;344:1343–50.

121. Knowler WC, Barrett-Connor E, Fowler SE et al. Reduction in the incidence of type 2 diabetes with lifestyle intervention or metformin. *N Engl J Med* 2002;346:393–403.

122. Batty GD, Lee IM. Physical activity and coronary heart disease. *BMJ* 2004;328:1089–90.

123. Astrup A, Meinert Larsen T, Harper A. Atkins and other low-carbohydrate diets: hoax or an effective tool for weight loss? *Lancet* 2004;364:897–9.

124. Padwal R, Li SK, Lau DC. Long-term pharmacotherapy for obesity and overweight. *Cochrane Database Syst Rev* 2004(3):CD004094.

125. Torgerson JS, Hauptman J, Boldrin MN et al. XENical in the prevention of diabetes in obese subjects (XENDOS) study: a randomized study of orlistat as an adjunct to lifestyle changes for the prevention of type 2 diabetes in obese patients. *Diabetes Care* 2004;27:155–61.

126. Buchwald H, Avidor Y, Braunwald E, et al. Bariatric surgery: a systematic review and meta-analysis. *JAMA* 2004;292:1724–37.

127. Black SC. Cannabinoid receptor antagonists and obesity. *Curr Opin Investig Drugs* 2004;5:389–94.

128. The Diabetes Control and Complications Trial Research Group. The effect of intensive treatment of diabetes on the development and progression of long-term complications in insulin-dependent diabetes mellitus. *N Engl J Med* 1993;329:977–86.

129. UK Prospective Diabetes Study (UKPDS) Group. Intensive blood-glucose control with sulphonylureas or insulin compared with conventional treatment and risk of complications in patients with type 2 diabetes (UKPDS 33). *Lancet* 1998;352:837–53.

130. Nathan DM, Lachin J, Cleary P et al. Intensive diabetes therapy and carotid intima-media thickness in type 1 diabetes mellitus. *N Engl J Med* 2003;348:2294–303.

131. Larsen JL, Colling CW, Ratanasuwan T et al. Pancreas transplantation improves vascular disease in patients with type 1 diabetes. *Diabetes Care* 2004;27:1706–11.

132. Navarro X, Kennedy WR, Sutherland DE. Autonomic neuropathy

and survival in diabetes mellitus: effects of pancreas transplantation. *Diabetologia* 1991;34 (Suppl 1):S108–12.

133. Krentz AJ. Sulfonylureas in the prevention of cardiovascular disease: from UGDP to the ADVANCE study. Padua: VIII european symposium on metabolism 2003, 261–77.

134. Gribble FM, Reimann F. Pharmacological modulation of K(ATP) channels. *Biochem Soc Trans* 2002;30:333–9.

135. Huizar JF, Gonzalez LA, Alderman J et al. Sulfonylureas attenuate electrocardiographic ST-segment elevation during an acute myocardial infarction in diabetics. *J Am Coll Cardiol* 2003;42:1017–21.

136. Gaede P, Vedel P, Larsen N et al. Multifactorial intervention and cardiovascular disease in patients with type 2 diabetes. *N Engl J Med* 2003;348:383–93.

137. Stratton IM, Adler AI, Neil HA et al. Association of glycaemia with macrovascular and microvascular complications of type 2 diabetes (UKPDS 35): prospective observational study. *BMJ* 2000;321:405–12.

138. Krentz AJ. UKPDS and beyond: into the next millennium. United Kingdom Prospective Diabetes Study. *Diabetes Obes Metab* 1999;1:13–22.

139. Olsson J, Lindberg G, Gottsater M et al. Increased mortality in Type II diabetic patients using sulphonylurea and metformin in combination: a population-based observational study. *Diabetologia* 2000;43:558–60.

140. Krentz AJ, Bailey CJ. Type 2 diabetes in practice. London: Royal Society of Medicine Press, 2001.

141. Lalau JD, Race JM. Lactic acidosis in metformin therapy: searching for a link with metformin in reports of 'metformin-associated lactic acidosis'. *Diabetes Obes Metab* 2001;3:195–201.

142. Krentz AJ, Bailey CJ, Melander A. Thiazolidinediones for type 2 diabetes. New agents reduce insulin resistance but need long term clinical trials. *BMJ* 2000;321:252–3.

143. Day C. Thiazolidinediones: a new class of antidiabetic drugs. *Diabet Med* 1999;16:179–92.

144. Martens FM, Visseren FL, Lemay J et al. Metabolic and additional vascular effects of thiazolidinediones. *Drugs* 2002;62:1463–80.

145. Yki-Jarvinen H. Thiazolidinediones. *N Engl J Med* 2004;351:1106–18.

146. Nesto RW, Bell D, Bonow RO et al. Thiazolidinedione use, fluid retention, and congestive heart failure: a consensus statement from the American Heart Association and American Diabetes

Association. October 7, 2003. *Circulation* 2003;108:2941–8.

147. Capes SE, Hunt D, Malmberg K et al. Stress hyperglycaemia and increased risk of death after myocardial infarction in patients with and without diabetes: a systematic overview. *Lancet* 2000;355:773–8.

148. Stevens RJ, Coleman RL, Adler AI et al. Risk factors for myocardial infarction case fatality and stroke case fatality in type 2 diabetes: UKPDS 66. *Diabetes Care* 2004;27:201–7.

149. Norhammar A, Tenerz A, Nilsson G et al. Glucose metabolism in patients with acute myocardial infarction and no previous diagnosis of diabetes mellitus: a prospective study. *Lancet* 2002;359:2140–4.

150. Malmberg K. Prospective randomised study of intensive insulin treatment on long term survival after acute myocardial infarction in patients with diabetes mellitus. DIGAMI (Diabetes Mellitus, Insulin Glucose Infusion in Acute Myocardial Infarction) Study Group. *BMJ* 1997;314:1512–5.

151. Malmberg K, Ryden L, Wedel H, et al. Intense metabolic control by means of insulin in patients with diabetes mellitus and acute myocardial infarction (DIGAMI 2). *Eur Heart J* 2005;26:650–61.

152. Opie LH. Proof that glucose-insulin-potassium provides metabolic protection of ischaemic myocardium? *Lancet* 1999;353:768 9.

153. Iozzo P, Chareonthaitawee P, Dutka D et al. Independent association of type 2 diabetes and coronary artery disease with myocardial insulin resistance. *Diabetes* 2002;51:3020–4.

154. Vijan S, Hayward RA. Pharmacologic lipid-lowering therapy in type 2 diabetes mellitus: background paper for the American College of Physicians. *Ann Intern Med* 2004;140:650–8.

155. Manley SE, Stratton IM, Cull CA et al. Effects of three months' diet after diagnosis of Type 2 diabetes on plasma lipids and lipoproteins (UKPDS 45). UK Prospective Diabetes Study Group. *Diabet Med* 2000;17:518–23.

156. Efficacy of atenolol and captopril in reducing risk of macrovascular and microvascular complications in type 2 diabetes: UKPDS 39. UK Prospective Diabetes Study Group. *BMJ* 1998;317:713–20.

157. Kuller LH. Hormone replacement therapy and risk of cardiovascular disease: implications of the results of the Women's Health Initiative. *Arterioscler Thromb Vasc Biol* 2003;23:11–6.

158. Randomised trial of cholesterol lowering in 4444 patients with coronary heart disease: the Scandinavian Simvastatin Survival Study (4S). *Lancet* 1994;344:1383–9.

159. Sacks FM, Pfeffer MA, Moye LA et al. The effect of pravastatin on coronary events after myocardial infarction in patients with average cholesterol levels. Cholesterol and Recurrent Events Trial

investigators. *N Engl J Med* 1996;335:1001–9.

160. Haffner SM. The Scandinavian Simvastatin Survival Study (4S) subgroup analysis of diabetic subjects: implications for the prevention of coronary heart disease. *Diabetes Care* 1997;20:469–71.

161. Goldberg RB, Mellies MJ, Sacks FM et al. Cardiovascular events and their reduction with pravastatin in diabetic and glucose-intolerant myocardial infarction survivors with average cholesterol levels: subgroup analyses in the cholesterol and recurrent events (CARE) trial. The Care Investigators. *Circulation* 1998;98:2513–9.

162. MRC/BHF Heart Protection Study of cholesterol lowering with simvastatin in 20,536 high-risk individuals: a randomised placebo-controlled trial. *Lancet* 2002;360:7–22.

163. Collins R, Armitage J, Parish S et al. MRC/BHF Heart Protection Study of cholesterol-lowering with simvastatin in 5963 people with diabetes: a randomised placebo-controlled trial. *Lancet* 2003;361:2005–16.

164. MRC/BHF Heart Protection Study of antioxidant vitamin supplementation in 20,536 high-risk individuals: a randomised placebo-controlled trial. *Lancet* 2002;360:23–33.

165. The ALLHAT Officers and Coordinators for the ALLHAT Collaborative Research Group. Major outcomes in moderately hypercholesterolemic, hypertensive patients randomized to pravastatin vs usual care: The Antihypertensive and Lipid-Lowering Treatment to Prevent Heart Attack Trial (ALLHAT–LLT). *JAMA* 2002;288:2998–3007.

166. Sever PS, Dahlof B, Poulter NR et al. Prevention of coronary and stroke events with atorvastatin in hypertensive patients who have average or lower-than-average cholesterol concentrations, in the Anglo–Scandinavian Cardiac Outcomes Trial–Lipid Lowering Arm (ASCOT–LLA): a multicentre randomised controlled trial. *Lancet* 2003;361:1149–58.

167. Colhoun HM, Betteridge DJ, Durrington PN et al. Primary prevention of cardiovascular disease with atorvastatin in type 2 diabetes in the Collaborative Atorvastatin Diabetes Study (CARDS): multicentre randomised placebo-controlled trial. *Lancet* 2004;364:685–96.

168. Temelkova-Kurktschiev T, Hanefeld M. The lipid triad in type 2 diabetes – prevalence and relevance of hypertriglyceridaemia/low high-density lipoprotein syndrome in type 2 diabetes. *Exp Clin Endocrinol Diabetes* 2004;112:75–9.

169. Koskinen P, Manttari M, Manninen V et al. Coronary heart disease incidence in NIDDM patients in the Helsinki Heart

Study. *Diabetes Care* 1992;15:820–5.

170. Manninen V, Tenkanen L, Koskinen P et al. Joint effects of serum triglyceride and LDL cholesterol and HDL cholesterol concentrations on coronary heart disease risk in the Helsinki Heart Study. Implications for treatment. *Circulation* 1992;85:37–45.

171. Rubins HB, Robins SJ, Collins D et al. Gemfibrozil for the secondary prevention of coronary heart disease in men with low levels of high-density lipoprotein cholesterol. Veterans Affairs High-Density Lipoprotein Cholesterol Intervention Trial Study Group. *N Engl J Med* 1999;341:410–8.

172. Robins SJ, Rubins HB, Faas FH et al. Insulin resistance and cardiovascular events with low HDL cholesterol: the Veterans Affairs HDL Intervention Trial (VA–HIT). *Diabetes Care* 2003;26:1513–7.

173. Diabetes Atherosclerosis Intervention Study Investigators. Effect of fenofibrate on progression of coronary-artery disease in type 2 diabetes: the Diabetes Atherosclerosis Intervention Study, a randomised study. *Lancet* 2001;357:905–10.

174. Williams B, Poulter NR, Brown MJ et al. British Hypertension Society guidelines for hypertension management 2004 (BHS–IV): summary. *BMJ* 2004;328:634 40.

175. Grundy SM, Cleeman JI, Merz CN et al. Implications of recent clinical trials for the National Cholesterol Education Program Adult Treatment Panel III guidelines. *Circulation* 2004;110:227–39.

176. Association AD. Summary of revisions for the 2005 practice recommendations. *Diabetes Care* 2005;28(Suppl 1):S3.

177. Nissen SE. High-dose statins in acute coronary syndromes: not just lipid levels. *JAMA* 2004;292:1365–7.

178. Ehrenstein MR, Jury EC, Mauri C. Statins for atherosclerosis—as good as it gets? *N Engl J Med* 2005;352:73–5.

179. Davidson MH, Toth PP. Combination therapy in the management of complex dyslipidemias. *Curr Opin Lipidol* 2004;15:423–31.

180. Bianchi S, Bigazzi R, Caiazza A et al. A controlled, prospective study of the effects of atorvastatin on proteinuria and progression of kidney disease. *Am J Kidney Dis* 2003;41:565–70.

181. Cannon CP, Braunwald E, McCabe CH et al. Intensive versus moderate lipid lowering with statins after acute coronary syndromes. *N Engl J Med* 2004;350:1495–504.

182. Schwartz GG, Olsson AG, Ezekowitz MD et al. Effects of atorvastatin on early recurrent ischemic events in acute coronary syndromes: the MIRACL study: a randomized controlled trial. *JAMA* 2001;285:1711–8.

183. Alsheikh-Ali AA, Kuvin JT, Karas RH. Risk of adverse events with fibrates. *Am J Cardiol* 2004;94:935–8.

184. Evans M, Roberts A, Davies S. Medical lipid-regulating therapy: current evidence, ongoing trials and future developments. *Drugs* 2004;64:1181–96.

185. van der Steeg W, Kuivenhoven J, Klerkx A et al. Role of CETP inhibitors in the treatment of dyslipidemia. *Curr Opin Lipidol* 2004;15:631–6.

186. Thompson GR. Is good cholesterol always good? *BMJ* 2004;329:471–2.

187. Brousseau ME, Schaefer EJ, Wolfe ML et al. Effects of an inhibitor of cholesteryl ester transfer protein on HDL cholesterol. *N Engl J Med* 2004;350:1505–15.

188. Bhatnagar D, Durrington PN. Omega-3 fatty acids: their role in the prevention and treatment of atherosclerosis related risk factors and complications. *Int J Clin Pract* 2003;57:305–14.

189. Curb JD, Pressel SL, Cutler JA et al. Effect of diuretic-based antihypertensive treatment on cardiovascular disease risk in older diabetic patients with isolated systolic hypertension. Systolic Hypertension in the Elderly Program Cooperative Research Group. *JAMA* 1996;276:1886–92.

190. Staessen JA, Fagard R, Thijs L et al. Randomised double-blind comparison of placebo and active treatment for older patients with isolated systolic hypertension. The Systolic Hypertension in Europe (Syst–Eur) Trial Investigators. *Lancet* 1997;350:757–64.

191. Tight blood pressure control and risk of macrovascular and microvascular complications in type 2 diabetes: UKPDS 38. UK Prospective Diabetes Study Group. *BMJ* 1998;317:703–13.

192. Hansson L, Zanchetti A, Carruthers SG et al. Effects of intensive blood-pressure lowering and low-dose aspirin in patients with hypertension: principal results of the Hypertension Optimal Treatment (HOT) randomised trial. HOT Study Group. *Lancet* 1998;351:1755–62.

193. Major outcomes in high-risk hypertensive patients randomized to angiotensin-converting enzyme inhibitor or calcium channel blocker vs diuretic: The Antihypertensive and Lipid-Lowering Treatment to Prevent Heart Attack Trial (ALLHAT). *JAMA* 2002;288:2981–97.

194. Yusuf S, Sleight P, Pogue J et al. Effects of an angiotensin-converting-enzyme inhibitor, ramipril, on cardiovascular events in high-risk patients. The Heart Outcomes Prevention Evaluation Study Investigators. *N Engl J Med* 2000;342:145–53.

195. Effects of ramipril on cardiovascular and microvascular outcomes

in people with diabetes mellitus: results of the HOPE study and MICRO–HOPE substudy. Heart Outcomes Prevention Evaluation Study Investigators. *Lancet* 2000;355:253–9.

196. Lindholm LH, Ibsen H, Dahlof B et al. Cardiovascular morbidity and mortality in patients with diabetes in the Losartan Intervention For Endpoint reduction in hypertension study (LIFE): a randomised trial against atenolol. *Lancet* 2002;359:1004–10.

197. Fox KM. Efficacy of perindopril in reduction of cardiovascular events among patients with stable coronary artery disease: randomised, double-blind, placebo-controlled, multicentre trial (the EUROPA study). *Lancet* 2003;362:782–8.

198. Braunwald E, Domanski MJ, Fowler SE et al for the PEACE trial investigators. Angiotensin-converting-enzyme inhibition in stable coronary artery disease. *N Engl J Med* 2004;351:2058–68.

199. Pitt B. ACE inhibitors for patients with vascular disease without left ventricular dysfunction – May they rest in PEACE? *N Engl J Med* 2004;351:2115–7.

200. Barnett AH, Bain SC, Bouter P et al. Angiotensin-receptor blockade versus converting-enzyme inhibition in type 2 diabetes and nephropathy. *N Engl J Med* 2004;351:1952–61.

201. Ruggenenti P, Fassi A, Ilieva AP et al. Preventing microalbuminuria in type 2 diabetes. *N Engl J Med* 2004;351: 1941–51.

202. Remuzzi G, Chiurchiu C, Ruggenenti P. Proteinuria predicting outcome in renal disease: Nondiabetic nephropathies (REIN). *Kidney Int Suppl* 2004:S90–6.

203. Scheen AJ. Prevention of type 2 diabetes mellitus through inhibition of the renin-angiotensin system. *Drugs* 2004;64: 2537–65.

204. Sowers JR. Insulin resistance and hypertension. *Am J Physiol Heart Circ Physiol* 2004;286:H1597–602.

205. Gress TW, Nieto FJ, Shahar E et al. Hypertension and antihypertensive therapy as risk factors for type 2 diabetes mellitus. Atherosclerosis Risk in Communities Study. *N Engl J Med* 2000;342:905–12.

206. Verdecchia P, Reboldi G, Angeli F et al. Adverse prognostic significance of new diabetes in treated hypertensive subjects. *Hypertension* 2004;43:963–9.

207. Krentz AJ, Evans AJ. Selective imidazoline receptor agonists for metabolic syndrome. *Lancet* 1998;351:152–3.

208. Bakris GL. Hypertension and nephropathy. *Am J Med* 2003;115(Suppl 8A):49S–54S.

209. Association AD. Hypertension management in adults with diabetes. *Diabetes Care* 2004;27:s65–s67.
210. Moreno PR, Murcia AM, Palacios IF et al. Coronary composition and macrophage infiltration in atherectomy specimens from patients with diabetes mellitus. *Circulation* 2000;102:2180–4.
211. Otter W, Kleybrink S, Doering W et al. Hospital outcome of acute myocardial infarction in patients with and without diabetes mellitus. *Diabet Med* 2004;21:183–7.
212. Mak KH, Moliterno DJ, Granger CB et al. Influence of diabetes mellitus on clinical outcome in the thrombolytic era of acute myocardial infarction. GUSTO–I Investigators. Global Utilization of Streptokinase and Tissue Plasminogen Activator for Occluded Coronary Arteries. *J Am Coll Cardiol* 1997;30: 171–9.
213. Veglio M, Chinaglia A, Cavallo-Perin P. QT interval, cardiovascular risk factors and risk of death in diabetes. *J Endocrinol Invest* 2004;27:175–81.
214. Pfeffer MA, McMurray JJ, Velazquez EJ et al. Valsartan, captopril, or both in myocardial infarction complicated by heart failure, left ventricular dysfunction, or both. *N Engl J Med* 2003;349:1893–906.
215. Antiplatelet Trialists' Collaboration. Collaborative overview of randomised trials of antiplatelet therapy. I: Prevention of death, myocardial infarction, and stroke by prolonged antiplatelet therapy in various categories of patients. *BMJ* 1994;308:81–106.
216. Steering Committee of the Physicians' Health Study Research Group. Final report on the aspirin component of the ongoing Physicians' Health Study. *N Engl J Med* 1989;321:129–35.
217. Early Treatment Diabetic Retinopathy Study Investigators. Aspirin effects on mortality and morbidity in patients with diabetes mellitus. Early Treatment Diabetic Retinopathy Study report 14. *JAMA* 1992;268:1292–300.
218. American Diabetes Association. Aspirin therapy in diabetes. *Diabetes Care* 2004;27:s72–s73.
219. Colwell JA. Antiplatelet agents for the prevention of cardiovascular disease in diabetes mellitus. *Am J Cardiovasc Drugs* 2004;4:87–106.
220. Beatt KJ, Morgan KP, Kapur A. Revascularisation in diabetics with multivessel coronary artery disease. *Heart* 2004;90:999–1002.
221. Bell DS. Heart failure: the frequent, forgotten, and often fatal complication of diabetes. *Diabetes Care* 2003;26:2433–41.

222. Kannel WB, McGee DL. Diabetes and cardiovascular disease. The Framingham study. *JAMA* 1979;241:2035–8.

223. Malmberg K, Ryden L, Efendic S et al. Randomized trial of insulin-glucose infusion followed by subcutaneous insulin treatment in diabetic patients with acute myocardial infarction (DIGAMI study): effects on mortality at 1 year. *J Am Coll Cardiol* 1995;26: 57–65.

224. Kenchaiah S, Evans JC, Levy D et al. Obesity and the risk of heart failure. *N Engl J Med* 2002;347:305–13.

225. Bruno G, Giunti S, Bargero G et al. Sex-differences in prevalence of electrocardiographic left ventricular hypertrophy in Type 2 diabetes: the Casale Monferrato Study. *Diabet Med* 2004;21:823–8.

226. Zile MR, Baicu CF, Gaasch WH. Diastolic heart failure— abnormalities in active relaxation and passive stiffness of the left ventricle. *N Engl J Med* 2004;350:1953–9.

227. Wang TJ, Larson MG, Levy D et al. Plasma natriuretic peptide levels and the risk of cardiovascular events and death. *N Engl J Med* 2004;350:655–63.

228. Bhalla MA, Chiang A, Epshteyn VA et al. Prognostic role of B-type natriuretic peptide levels in patients with type 2 diabetes mellitus. *J Am Coll Cardiol* 2004;44:1047–52.

229. Jessup M, Brozena S. Heart failure. *N Engl J Med* 2003;348: 2007–18.

230. Pfeffer MA, Swedberg K, Granger CB et al. Effects of candesartan on mortality and morbidity in patients with chronic heart failure: the CHARM–Overall programme. *Lancet* 2003;362:759–66.

231. White HD. Candesartan and heart failure: the allure of CHARM. *Lancet* 2003;362:754–5.

232. Pitt B, Remme W, Zannad F et al. Eplerenone, a selective aldosterone blocker, in patients with left ventricular dysfunction after myocardial infarction. *N Engl J Med* 2003;348:1309–21.

233. Packer M, Bristow MR, Cohn JN et al. The effect of carvedilol on morbidity and mortality in patients with chronic heart failure. U.S. Carvedilol Heart Failure Study Group. *N Engl J Med* 1996;334:1349–55.

234. Capes SE, Hunt D, Malmberg K. Stress hyperglycemia and prognosis of stroke in nondiabetic and diabetic patients: a systematic overview. *Stroke* 2001;32:2426–32.

235. Levetan CS. Effect of hyperglycemia on stroke outcomes. *Endocr Pract* 2004;10 (Suppl 2):34–9.

236. Catto AJ, Grant PJ. Risk factors for cerebrovascular disease and the role of coagulation and fibrinolysis. *Blood Coagul Fibrinolysis* 1995;6:497–510.

237. Watson GS, Craft S. Modulation of memory by insulin and glucose: neuropsychological observations in Alzheimer's disease. *Eur J Pharmacol* 2004;490:97–113.

238. Cryer PE. Diverse causes of hypoglycemia–associated autonomic failure in diabetes. *N Engl J Med* 2004;350:2272–9.

239. Yaffe K, Blackwell T, Kanaya AM et al. Diabetes, impaired fasting glucose, and development of cognitive impairment in older women. *Neurology* 2004;63:658–63.

240. Messier C. Diabetes, Alzheimer's disease and apolipoprotein genotype. *Exp Gerontol* 2003;38:941–6.

241. Luchsinger JA, Tang MX, Shea S et al. Hyperinsulinemia and risk of Alzheimer disease. *Neurology* 2004;63:1187–92.

242. Haan MN, Wallace R. Can dementia be prevented? Brain aging in a population-based context. *Ann Rev Public Health* 2004;25: 1–24.

243. Aronow WS, Frishman WH. Treatment of hypertension and prevention of ischemic stroke. *Curr Cardiol Rep* 2004;6:124–9.

244. Albers GW, Amarenco P, Easton JD et al. Antithrombotic and thrombolytic therapy for ischemic stroke: the Seventh ACCP Conference on Antithrombotic and Thrombolytic Therapy. *Chest* 2004;126(3 Suppl):483S–512S.

245. Collins R, Armitage J, Parish S et al. Effects of cholesterol-lowering with simvastatin on stroke and other major vascular events in 20536 people with cerebrovascular disease or other high-risk conditions. *Lancet* 2004;363:757–67.

246. Rothwell PM, Eliasziw M, Gutnikov SA et al. Endarterectomy for symptomatic carotid stenosis in relation to clinical subgroups and timing of surgery. *Lancet* 2004;363:915–24.

247. Selvin E, Erlinger TP. Prevalence of and risk factors for peripheral arterial disease in the United States: results from the National Health and Nutrition Examination Survey, 1999–2000. *Circulation* 2004;110:738–43.

248. Adler AI, Stevens RJ, Neil A et al. UKPDS 59: hyperglycemia and other potentially modifiable risk factors for peripheral vascular disease in type 2 diabetes. *Diabetes Care* 2002;25:894–9.

249. Brass EP, Hiatt WR. Acquired skeletal muscle metabolic myopathy in atherosclerotic peripheral arterial disease. *Vasc Med* 2000;5:55–9.

250. American Diabetes Association. Peripheral arterial disease in people with diabetes. *Diabetes Care* 2003;26:3333–41.

251. CAPRIE Steering Committee. A randomised, blinded, trial of clopidogrel versus aspirin in patients at risk of ischaemic events (CAPRIE). *Lancet* 1996;348:1329–39.

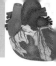

252. Burns P, Gough S, Bradbury AW. Management of peripheral arterial disease in primary care. *BMJ* 2003;326:584–8.

253. Mohler ER. The effect of risk factor changes on peripheral arterial disease and cardiovascular risk. *Curr Drug Targets Cardiovasc Haematol Disord* 2004;4:259–63.

254. Jacoby D, Mohler ER. Drug treatment of intermittent claudication. *Drugs* 2004;64:1657–70.

255. Krentz AJ, Bailey CJ. Type 2 diabetes in practice (2nd edition). London: Royal Society of Medicine Press, 2005.

256. Fox CS, Coady S, Sorlie PD et al. Trends in cardiovascular complications of diabetes. *JAMA* 2004;292:2495–9.

257. Bryer-Ash M, Garber AJ. Inpatient glucose management: the emperor finally has clothes. *Diabetes Care* 2005;28:973–5.

INDEX

Notes: all entries refer to diabetes and cardiovascular disease unless otherwise stated. Page numbers in *italics* denote figures and tables. Abbreviations, CVD = cardiovascular disease.

157

prevention, 65–66
hypertension, 51
insulin resistance, 30–31
lipids, 49, *50*
    abnormalities, *50*
microalbuminuria, 55
type 2 diabetes
apolipoprotein B, 48–49
children/adolescents, 11
diagnosis, *37*
diet, 61–63
dyslipidaemia pattern, 45–46
glycaemic control, 44
hyperglycaemia, 33
    treatment/prevention, 65, *66*,
    66–72
    see also specific drugs
hypertension, 50, 53
insulin resistance, 26
lipid abnormalities, *50*
microalbuminuria, 55
polycystic ovary syndrome, 26
prevention, 61–63, *62*
statins, 16
vascular function, 30

U

Ultratard, 131
United Kingdom Prospective
    Diabetes Study (UKPDS), 16, 65,
    68
cerebrovascular disease, 102
heart failure, 100–101
hypertension, 84–86, *85*, 94
metformin, *70*, 113, 114
peripheral artery disease, 105, 108
urinalysis, 54

V

valsartan, 98, 102
vascular autoregulation
    impairment, 52

vascular cell adhesion molecule-1
    (VCAM-1), 35
vascular damage in hyperglycaemia,
    34–36
very-low-density lipoprotein (VLDL)
    apolipoprotein B role in secretion,
    48
glycaemic control, 44
hepatic synthesis in type 2
diabetes, 45–46, *46*
insulin resistance effects, *47*
Veterans Administration High
    Density lipoprotein Intervention
    Trial (VA-HIT), 80
visceral fat accumulation, 24
voglibose, 129

W

waist circumference, 22–23
warfarin, 82, 104
websites, 135–136
weight loss
    hypertension, 91
    polycystic ovary syndrome, 26
    type 2 diabetes prevention, 61
'white coat' hypertension, 54
Whitehall study, 39
whole body insulin resistance/
    sensitivity
    heart failure risk, 100
    thiazolidinediones, 70–71
women, CVD risk, 12–13, *13*
Women's Health Initiative
    (WHI), 13
Women's Health Study, 59
World Health Organization, 21

X

xanthomata, 49

Z

zidovudine, 65